HEALTH & BEAUTY HANDBOOK

Susan Kerr

TEACH YOURSELF BOOKS

This book is dedicated to my daughter Katie

Acknowledgements

I would like to thank Stephanie Henderson for her beauty insider insights, Dr Richard Maxwell MA FRCGP for his health overview and Cheryl Scott and Gabriella Zuckerman for their cosmetic chemists' review. Also Anne Waldman, Director of Writing and Poetics at The Naropa Institute for permission to print part of her poem, Alexander Kerr for his championship and Michael Kerr for his love and his family and critical skills.

The author and publisher would like to thank IPC Magazines for their kind permission to reproduce the photographs which were first published in *Essentials* Magazine.

Long-renowned as the authoritative source for self-guided learning – with more than 30 million copies sold worldwide – the *Teach Yourself* series includes over 200 titles in the fields of languages, crafts, hobbies, sports, and other leisure activities.

Library of Congress Catalog Card Number: on file

First published in UK 1997 by Hodder Headline Plc, 338 Euston Road, London NW1 3BH

A catalogue record for this title is available from the British Library.

First published in US 1997 by NTC Publishing Group, 4255 West Touhy Avenue, Lincolnwood (Chicago), Illinois 60646 – 19975 U.S.A.

The 'Teach Yourself' name and logo are registered trade marks of Hodder & Stoughton Ltd in the UK.

Copyright © 1997 Susan Kerr

In UK: All rights reserved. No part of this publication may be reproduced or transmitted in any form or by any means, electronic or mechanical, including photocopy, recording, or any information storage and retrieval system, without permission in writing from the publisher or under licence from the Copyright Licensing Agency Limited. Further details of such licences (for reprographic reproduction) may be obtained from the Copyright Licensing Agency Limited, of 90 Tottenham Court Road, London W1P 9HE

In US: All rights reserved. No part of this book may be reproduced, stored in a retrieval system, or transmitted in any form, or by any means, electronic, mechanical, photocopying, or otherwise, without prior permission of NTC Publishing Group.

Typeset by Transet Limited, Coventry, England.

Printed in Great Britain by Cox & Wyman Limited, Reading, Berkshire.

Impression number 10 9 8 7 6 5 4 3 2 1
Year   2000 1999 1998 1997

CONTENTS

1 The Powerhouse of Beauty: Your Body — 5
 Six-step self-assessment: what body type are you? — 5
 Your own before-into-after plan — 9
 Powerhouse know-how: the heart of the matter — 10

2 Fuelling Your Powerhouse: Healthy Eating — 15
 Seven basic nutrients: eating for beauty — 15
 Ease into better eating — 18
 Nutrition tricks and timing — 19
 Predictable patterns of progress (or not) — 24

3 Energising Your Powerhouse: Exercise — 26
 Ease into exercise — 26
 How muscles work — 28
 Seven exercise routes — 29

4 Putting Your Best Face Forward: Skin — 38
 Two-part self-assessment: what's your skin type? — 38
 Skin know-how — 40
 Skincare product lowdown — 43
 Your steps to good-looking skin — 44
 Skincare specifics — 50
 Home-based skincare recipes — 54
 Making faces: complexion exercises — 55
 What a professional can do for you — 56

5 The Shining: Hair — 57
 Ten-step self-assessment: what's your hair profile? — 57
 Hair know-how: what is hair? — 59
 Haircare product lowdown — 63
 Your steps to good-looking hair — 64
 Haircare specifics — 67
 Do-it-yourself, no-hype haircare — 69
 Hair alive: hair exercises — 70

6 Essential You: Developing Personal Style — 72
 Colour me 'me': what's your season? — 72
 Style tips on body types: ten-step self-assessment — 76
 Style directions: attitude in action — 81
 Your own before-into-after style plan — 84

7	**Hair: Your Most Flexible Beauty Asset**	**90**
	Four-part self-assessment: what hairstyle for you?	90
	To the hairdresser: the cut is all	94
	Styling at home	97
	Perming and colouring	100
	Hairstyle on a budget, in a hurry	106
8	**Making Up: From Minimal to Dramatic**	**108**
	Five-stage self-assessment: what make-up style for you?	108
	Product lowdown: what make-up for whom?	109
	Colours for your skin, eyes and lips	115
	Your personal make-up style: step by step	118
	Bridal, portrait and television make-up	127
	What a professional can do	129
9	**Top to Toe: Total Bodycare**	**130**
	The nose knows: the art of fragrance	130
	A beautiful gesture: handcare	132
	On your toes: footcare	137
	Sleek and silky: skin all over	139
	Specific body problem areas	140
	Tan fantastic	142
10	**Your Wellspring of Wellbeing: Body, Soul and Self**	**146**
	Stress survival	146
	A system to beat illness and toxins	148
	Ages and stages: hormones, health and looks	149
	Women's health matters	153
	Your own de-stress plan	156
	Body and self wellbeing	159
11	**Professional and Medical Beauty Intervention**	**161**
	A beautiful smile: cosmetic dentistry	161
	Cosmetic surgery: the lowdown	163
	Permanent body decoration: piercing, tattoos, make-up	170
12	**Inside the Beauty Business**	**173**
	How a product is born	173
	Confronting beauty issues	176
	Product lowdown: a glossary of ingredients	181
	Beauty futures	183
	Resources	**186**
	Index	**188**

INTRODUCTION

> ❛ I am putting makeup on empty space
> all patinas convening on empty space
> rouge blushing on empty space
> I am putting makeup on empty space
> pasting eyelashes on empty space
> painting the eyebrows of empty space
> piling creams on empty space
> painting the phenomenal world ❜
>
> from *Makeup on Empty Space* by Anne Waldman

Every day almost everyone wakes up, looks in the mirror and thinks: 'That's okay,' or 'Hmm, could be better,' or possibly 'Aaargh, I need help!' I have worked in the beauty world for 25 years, and doing something about these feelings is, in my opinion, what beauty is about.

Beauty means caring for yourself. Beauty means defining yourself. Beauty means making the most of what you've got. Beauty can also mean luxurious self-indulgence. The kind of beauty that I describe in the pages of this book isn't impossible, perfect, magazine-model beauty, but possible, healthy, liveable, good-enough good looks. It's also your choice: your personal style.

Beauty is a business, too, a serious international, multibillion-dollar industry that touches your life – often your skin – every day. Its products enhance, its marketing persuades, its jargon and abundance of choices sometimes intimidate.

From my entré as Guest Beauty Editor of *Mademoiselle* magazine to my more recent work as a health writer and author – with stops at Coty, Revlon, Elizabeth Arden, Fashion Fair, Kanebo and other houses along the way – beauty has been about caring and about fun. It seems the time is right for an intelligent reader's beauty book, not just a how-to, but a how-it-works, for people who want to know more than just how to put on a lipstick. This *Teach Yourself Health and Beauty Handbook* aims to be down-to-earth, practical and helpful, to give you some of the tricks of the trade, to inform you with professional insight and to provide a few glimpses of the fascinating beauty business.

Beauty and guilt?

By now you've probably guessed that because beauty is about you as a real person, this book covers much more than make-up and hairstyles. I must pause here to deal with an issue that I've come to terms with; maybe you worry about it, too: is caring about your looks frivolous? On a world scale of things, I've decided, yes, it's frivolous. But on a 'you' scale of things, instinct insists – looks matter. It goes like this ...

What do you see when you look in a mirror? Your own self-image. This outer self is what the world sees of you. Is it really you? No, only part. But it is the part that the rest of the world knows first. It may seem wrong or unfair that the surface of you should matter so much, but it's been proven that a person makes a judgement of another person within seconds of meeting. It's not final, and it's not unchangeable, but it is a snap response based on a first impression. The reaction isn't verbal or even conscious, it's an attitude – a willingness to be open and receptive, or an inclination to be wary or negative. So it's not a harmful feminine trap or a vain waste of time and money to care about the surface of yourself – it's sound human nature.

Beyond outer impressions, beauty is far from frivolous because it includes the practical matter of personal comfort and hygiene. This is beauty as grooming: skin, hair, teeth, hands, feet, nails and body need to feel good and work well so that you can get on with being you. Here beauty clearly merges with health, for the state of your body is reflected in your looks.

INTRODUCTION

Good looks start here

Health is so important to beauty that this book begins with information and advice about the body, because if you know why you should do something, you're more likely to do it. Chapter 1, *The Powerhouse of Beauty: Your Body* explains the workings of the body systems that most affect skin, hair, nails and general appearance. Chapters 2 and 3 describe the food and maintenance true beauty requires.

With inner beauty on track, you can focus on the skin-deep aspects of looking good. Glossy hair and clear, glowing skin: these are the goals. Chapter 4, *Putting Your Best Face Forward: Skin*, and Chapter 5, *The Shining: Hair*, help you assess your skin and hair, inform you about their structure, care and maintenance. These chapters and others following give you the 'product lowdown', explaining the formulae and functions of beauty products on offer. You'll find do-it-yourself, home-made beauty recipes, too, and at the other extreme you'll find out what professional beauty experts can provide.

Back to the mirror

Hairstyles and make-up next? No, back to you, standing in front of your mirror, thinking about first impressions, your outer self. Your choice of haircut, hair colour, make-up and clothes is your arena for being *Essential You: Developing Personal Style*. Chapter 6 helps you to assess and use your physical strong points, identify your best colours, and to build on your own personality to find the magnetic true north of your own individual style.

With your options for personal style in mind, in Chapter 7, *Hair: Your Most Flexible Beauty Asset*, you'll learn how to talk your hairdresser's language, and consider your choices of colour, cut and curls (or not) to suit your own hair and your individual image. Naturally, make-up comes next, in Chapter 8, *Making Up: From Minimal to Dramatic*. What products should you use? What routines should you choose to make the most of your face, features and personal style?

Because healthy beauty doesn't stop at the neck, Chapter 9 addresses *Top to Toe: Total Bodycare*. Your hands and feet, the fragrance you wear, your skin from top to toe – there are a whole lot of 'how-to's for these beauty assets.

Chapter 10, *Your Wellspring of Wellbeing: Body, Soul and Self* reveals the whole-self secrets of healthy beauty, with insight into managing your stresses, immune system, hormones and general health. Because biology is a fact of life and looks, this chapter, and many others, contains 'Ages and Stages', a section with information of particular interest to women at particular times of life, from 14 to beyond 55.

But what if there's some part of your physical self that you really don't like? Something that make-up and healthy maintenance can't help? Chapter 11, *Professional and Medical Beauty Intervention*, considers cosmetic surgery and other qualified professional intervention for the sake of your looks. Some changes are reasonably easy to achieve, some are for fun, others are serious stuff; you have a right to plan a permanent change and you need the facts before you make your decision.

Inside story and happily ever after

Whether you are bewitched or bewildered by beauty products, you'll learn just what goes on *Inside the Beauty Business* in Chapter 12. It covers the birth of a beauty product and includes the lowdown on product testing, natural products and other issues. And if you're truly hooked on feeling good and looking good, perhaps you'd like to be a beauty insider yourself? Scan through the list of job descriptions and starting points – you can find a beauty career to meet your skills, interests, age and level of education.

Meanwhile, it's time to begin your own quest into healthy beauty and personal style. Self-assessments and achievable, before-into-after plans await. The mirror beckons. Does it say 'Okay', 'Hmmm...' or 'Help!'?

Note to readers

The ideas and practical suggestions in this book I offer as a writer and compiler of information. Neither I nor the publisher can accept responsibility for illness or injuries caused by a failure on the part of a reader to take professional cosmetic or medical advice.

1
THE POWERHOUSE OF BEAUTY: YOUR BODY

The twin pillars of true beauty are healthy eating and exercise. You can be flabby or living on junk food and still have style, so if you're content with this lifestyle you can skip everything before Chapter 6. However, it's an inescapable fact that really good health glows through in your looks: skin, hair, eyes, nails, bearing. And this kind of healthy natural beauty is not all that difficult to achieve.

What's the secret of getting yourself to believe in and act on what you know is good for you and your looks? I believe there are two main devices:

- Self-assessment and solid knowledge to support your motivation – What body type am I? How does my body work?
- Finding ways to eat and live healthily which painlessly fit your needs and lifestyle.

Further help, and confidence, comes from seeing yourself succeed at your own personal before-into-after plan.

Six-step self-assessment: What body type are you?

In a moment I'll ask you to go to a full-length mirror in privacy, pen and paper in hand. But first, a word about judging yourself. This is not an exercise in perfection. You do not even have to take off all your clothes. I'll bet you won't even do this right away, so after you've read this, as you go out to work, shop, collect the children, party or whatever, simply look at the people around you. Some are fat, some are lean, some older, younger, happy, stressed-out, smart, unkempt ... I dare say none is perfect, yet every one of them has something good about her or his looks. This is the background against which you should assess yourself, not magazine pages or the silver screen.

To get your feet firmly on the road to healthy beauty and personal style, write down your answers in this book or start a special notebook or journal.

Step 1   Height _____ (actual measurement)

Which description applies to you?

- Taller than most?
- Average to tall?
- Short to average?
- Shorter than most?

Now complete this sentence.

- I like/don't like my height because ...

There's not much you can do about your height, but your weight, bearing, clothes and confidence can all influence the overall impression. Practise positive thinking: tall women can call themselves model-like, stately, queenly, elegant; short women can see themselves as petite, delicate, vulnerable. It's fine if your personality doesn't match: there's a lot of mileage in the surprise of contrast.

Step 2   Bone structure and body type

Choose one word that describes you from each line.

- Shoulders are: narrow? well developed? rounded?
- Bones are: long? slender? average? sturdy? heavy?
- Build is: not curvy? athletic? soft?

The first words in each list describe ectomorphs, the middle words describe mesomorphs, the last are endomorphs. However, most people are a combination of these body types, so you might describe yourself as a meso-endomorph or an ecto-mesomorph. There's beauty in all types, from the lean-muscled thoroughbred to welcoming cuddly flesh.

THE POWERHOUSE OF BEAUTY: YOUR BODY

How difficult is it to change if you wish to? Generally, the metabolism of endomorphs is slower – they put on weight easily and find it harder to get it off. At the opposite extreme, ectomorphs tend to burn off calories quickly. Mesomorphs have a medium rate of metabolism. These tendencies give you a framework, but they are **not** an excuse to sit back and do nothing. Whatever your body type, diet and exercise can change your appearance.

Step 3 Weight _____ (actual weight)

Which of the following best describes your weight?

- Excellent for my height?
- Good to okay for my height?
- Wish it were less for my height?
- Overweight for my height?

Now complete this sentence.

- I'm happy/unhappy about my weight because ...

You'll find no height-and-weight charts here, they're too vague. Just use your eyes to judge if you're a 'good enough' weight. If you're happy with your weight, congratulations – as long as you didn't get there by taking diet pills, following extreme diets or indulging in binges. If you consider yourself okay-ish, you'd probably like to fine-tune your bodystyle patterns – most of us wish we could shed five pounds and tone up a bit. If you're overweight, are you simply plump? Lots of people like generous curves, so you can decide to tune up your health and lose a few pounds without worrying about getting radically thinner. If you are fat or obese, you can gradually work at getting your weight down, for a longer, fitter life if not for looks – it's best to consult your doctor and possibly Weight Watchers or a similar scheme for a long-term programme.

Step 4 Posture

You should wear minimal clothes or a leotard for this. You need views from front, back and side, standing, sitting and walking. Ask a friend to help or use a changing room three-way mirror, and check snapshots and videos of yourself. Circle descriptions that apply to you.

- **Head** (side view): thrusts forwards, chin lowered or raised? balanced on midline?

- **Neck**: scrunched? lengthened and aligned?
- **Shoulders**: rounded? hunched? uneven? level? open?
- **Back**: S-curve? concave or convex? straight spine?
- **Abdomen**: protruding? flat?
- **Bottom**: exaggerated protruding? gently rounded?
- **Arms**: thrown forwards or back? hang evenly relaxed?
- **Legs and knees**: rotated in or out? straight? facing forwards?
- **Weight distribution**: more on one foot and hip than the other? equally balanced between both sides?

Even a less than wonderful figure can look great with good body presentation. Clothes hang better and you look unmistakably confident. What's more, good posture patterns aid breathing, digestion, circulation and period problems. The first words in each line of the list above are postural flaws, the end words the ideal. If you notice any extreme flaws, especially in the back, knees or feet, it's best to see your doctor, an osteopath or an Alexander Technique teacher. Otherwise, fortunately, you can do something about almost any postural flaw you don't like. It's worth it – and not difficult – so try.

Step 5   Flab and fitness factor

- **Stomach, bottom, thighs, midriff, breasts, upper arm**: circle any of these that hang slack. Underline any that are firm and resilient.
- **Breathing**: Can you run for a bus and still be able to talk when you catch it? Do you, two or three times a week, exercise to the point where you get a little breathless? Or have you had no regular exercise recently? Have you never been out of breath since you left school? Have you never smoked? Are you an ex-smoker, or a smoker?
- **Flexibility**: Can you bend at the waist and touch your toes, sit on the floor and get up without using your hands, clean windows, reach high shelves, garden, bicycle, all without pain or stiffness?
- **Muscle strength**: Can you carry a weekender case or a full grocery bag several blocks, dig a 25-cm (10-inch) deep hole in garden soil, lift a toddler and carry her upstairs, each without stopping for a rest?

Too many negatives here means that your muscle tone needs work. Spot exercises, massage and certain beauty treatments can improve flabby parts of you. Whole-body exercises develop stamina, suppleness, breathing and strength. Can you do it? Yes. In Chapter 3 you'll find ways of getting fit to suit your personality and lifestyle.

Step 6 Age and stage

Are you:

- Under 16?
- 16–40?
- 40–55?
- Over 55?

Biology and life roles affect your good looks. Your hormones, especially if you're under 16 or in the 40 to 55 bracket, can wreak havoc on your weight, skin and hair. In the years from 16 to 40 looks and health may be affected by the demands of education, then career, and by the physical changes of childbirth and the demands of childcare. Over age 55, and sometimes as early as 40, time and gravity begin to show their effects. It's a fact that your basal metabolic rate (the rate at which you burn up energy in a totally calm resting state) decreases by about 5 per cent every 10 years – so weight builds up easily. Body systems and structure lose strength and elasticity if underused or misused. But you can take action against all these facts of life – specifics on what to do for ages and stages are given in Chapters 4, 6, 7, 8 and 10.

— Your own before-into-after plan —

So what's the verdict? Hopeless case? Never! There's a lot you can do to improve what you don't like; I promise you will see and feel genuine change, if you set out to try. But do not expect instant miracles. They're not good for you for three reasons. First, if you found an instant total miracle, like eliminating bags under your eyes, either it would be costly and probably painful or the effect would disappear just as instantly as it arrived. Second, the new you would feel a fake, and this would undermine your self-confidence. You need to grow gradually into a new you, to own and be pleased with the changes you have accomplished, so your confidence – the best-ever beauty asset – shines through. Third, your body as well as your self needs time to adapt to new ways. We're talking about building healthy beauty from cell level up, so it has a really secure foundation. Radical treatments, extreme diets or sudden hyper-exercise programmes destabilise and harm the body instead of helping.

To evolve into a better-looking you, take one small step at a time. Accept gracefully the things you can't change (height, body type, proportions, age). Query the things you can improve (posture, weight, tone and fitness, skin, hair and nail condition). Count your given blessings (big brown eyes, thick hair, shapely legs?). Note which things about you (proportions, features, clothes, make-up and hairstyle) you can accentuate or diminish.

Matters of style (clothes, hair, make-up, see Chapters 6, 7 and 8) you can effect fairly quickly. Matters of true healthy beauty begin here, and I'd suggest a realistic time frame of three months. Sounds too long? It's based on body fact; it takes approximately six months for your fingernail to grow from base to tip, two months for your hair to grow 1.25 cm ($1/2$ inch), and a month for your top layer of skin to renew itself. So it takes time to see the results of better eating and taking exercise. Think of it seasonally: first steps in winter, feel and see changes by spring, start in spring, see a difference by summer, and so forth. Working on this timescale your own before-into-after plan will gradually fine-tune your life patterns so that healthy beauty and style come naturally, without effort and without becoming obsessive. This is habit-forming health and good looks, based on the pleasure principle.

Powerhouse know-how: the heart of the matter

It may seem odd when we're talking about the bloom in your cheeks, the bounce in your hair and the length of your hemline, but it helps to know: your body systems have a huge influence on your surface image as well as your health. Any qualified health or beauty therapist is trained in physiology – the workings of the body systems. You, too, can be informed about the inner you and turn it to your beauty advantage. A bit of in-depth know-how is a great motivator, so we're now going to take a quick look at the major systems of the body. All interact, all are vital, but I'll start with the heart, a real workhorse.

THE POWERHOUSE OF BEAUTY: YOUR BODY

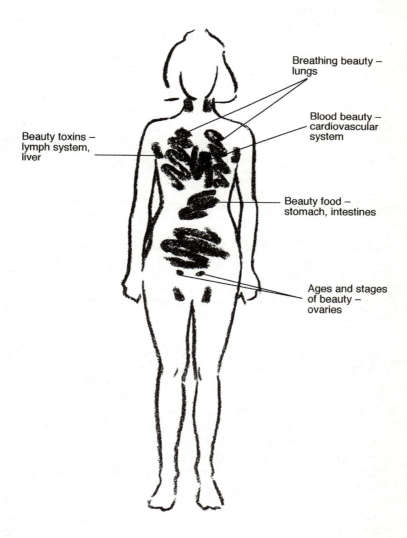

Figure 1 The powerhouse of beauty

Blood beauty

The cardiovascular (cardio = heart, vascular = veins/arteries) system circulates blood through your body thanks to your never-ceasing heart. From seven months before birth, the heart beats about 60 to 70 times every minute of every day. Sometimes it beats up to 200 times a minute. Why? The heart powers the blood transport system which delivers oxygen and nutrients to every cell in your body and carries away every cell's waste products. Blood circulation carries other elements, too: hormones and enzymes to trigger various body functions; platelets, white blood cells and antibodies to protect the body from infection and toxins. Blood also acts to regulate cell water content, body acid balance and body temperature.

So now you know: the heart pumps all the good stuff around your body and takes the bad stuff away. So good circulation means good skin, good hair, good nails, good everything.

Breathing beauty

The lungs bring oxygen into the body when you inhale and they get rid of oxygen's leftovers, carbon dioxide and water, when you exhale. Deep in the lungs the exchange of air takes place through tiny blood capillaries – here the respiratory system links into the cardiovascular system described above.

Why do you need oxygen? For the big E, energy. Not only energy for activities (running, talking, breathing, thinking, digesting, kissing) but also energy for growth and repair (in skin, for instance). Inside each body cell nutrients need oxygen for the chemical reaction that releases energy, a process called oxidation. It may not seem fair, but men and children oxidise food faster than women; even when they are sitting there doing nothing they burn up more calories. In other words, their metabolism is higher than women's. So you have to get plenty of oxygen circulating through your body to burn up food efficiently and to fuel life, looks and health.

Beauty food

From the mouth to the stomach to the large intestine and a few other places as well, the digestive system converts food into simple nutrient elements that can be carried into the blood. Digestion breaks down food physically and chemically, turning carbohydrates, fats and proteins into molecules cells can absorb. There's an amazing connection between your digestion and your brain. Just the thought (think lemon!) of food can start gastric juices flowing; the sight of food also triggers the process. Your brain and nervous system, interpreters as they are of your emotions, can have a big impact on how effectively your digestion works.

Obviously, quality of food counts for a lot (we'll come to that in Chapter 2), but you see now how the digestive, respiratory and cardiovascular systems interweave to supply every cell in the body with nutrients and oxygen for energy: heat, action, growth and repair.

Beauty toxins

One of the side effects of making energy is waste. The blood carries cell nutrient waste. The lungs excrete oxygen's waste, carbon dioxide and water. The bowels eliminate indigestible food parts and excess water. The kidneys and the skin's sweat glands get rid of water as well. The liver, among its other functions, destroys or de-arms toxic substances, such as drugs, chemicals, alcohol.

If your body is ineffective at eliminating waste, toxins can build up. The grapefruit-dimpling of cellulite is believed to be due to trapped toxins. Constipation and sluggish elimination can cause a harmful build up of toxins – seen as poor skin, felt as poor spirits, even as ill-health.

The rest of your powerhouse body beauty systems

There's still a lot more to the physiology of life, health and looks. The musculo-skeletal system (bones, joints, muscles) gives you structure and lets you move. The integumentary system (skin, nails, hair) provides protection and temperature regulation as well as the outer surface you see in the mirror. The nervous system (brain, spinal cord, nerves) sends and receives messages all over the body, both internally and via the sense organs (skin, nose, tongue, ears, eyes). Then there are the reproductive system and the endocrine system (hormones) – which influences many processes from instant (adrenalin danger alert) to long-term (rate and timing of growth). And finally there's the lymphatic system, a key part of the immune system. I'll cover some of these in more detail in later chapters, but there's one more stop before I conclude this body-beautiful tour.

Cell power

This is the micro-level of health and – ultimately – your whole appearance. Knowing about it may be just the life raft that will help you keep to healthy macro (life) patterns. Each cell in your body – each one of trillions – has an identity and a job to do. Inside each cell tiny structures order the cell's activities. To carry on efficiently, each single cell depends on its outer barrier, the cell membrane. This wall is thin, elastic and complex, made of proteins and lipids (fats). It has pores that allow water, oxygen, carbon dioxide, nutrients and waste in and out of the cell. Your skin is important for protecting and regulating your whole body; the cell membrane is important for each cell. So think when you're contemplating what to eat or whether to exercise, think of your cells, tiny but vitally powerful. A healthy cell is a healthy, great-looking you.

> It's incredibly intricate, your body – as you read this box wiggle your toes. Visualise your foot, its muscles contracting and relaxing, crossed by veins and arteries full of steadily-pumped blood, woven through with nerve endings giving you sensation and control, all made up of masses of individual living cells .... It's worth thinking about this miracle of a body every now and then, to motivate you to give it the diet, exercise and care that will result in better health and beauty for you.

2

FUELLING YOUR POWERHOUSE: HEALTHY EATING

As the computer jargon goes: garbage in, garbage out. Good nutrients are vital so that your trillion body cells can make up an energetic, good-looking you. Good diet how-tos and your own before-into-after plan follow soon in this chapter, but first we start with the basics. What exactly are good nutrients and how do they work for you?

Seven basic nutrients: eating for beauty

1 **Growth-power proteins**: build and repair body tissue. Sources are *meat, poultry, milk, eggs, fish, soya beans; lentils, pulses, nuts* also provide partial protein. Western diets include excessive protein; we need only about 60 g (2 oz) per day. The digestive process breaks protein into amino acids for cells to use.
2 **Energetic carbohydrates**: provide energy for activity and warmth. *Pasta, bread, cereals, potatoes, vegetables and fruits* contain starches that release energy slowly and satisfy hunger. *Sweet biscuits, cakes, chocolate bars, deserts, soft drinks and juices* are high in hunger-trigger sugars (see sugar tips below). The digestive process slowly breaks starches into a simple sugar, called glucose, for transport and use by cells. The body can make all the glucose it needs from starches; it does not need straight sugar, which the Western diet provides in abundance. Excess carbohydrates are stored by the body as fat.

THE HEALTH AND BEAUTY HANDBOOK

3 **Essential** (and not so) **fats**: protect organs, provide insulation, transport certain vitamins, provide energy. *Olive oil, sunflower and other vegetable oils, nuts and avocados* are examples of vegetable fat sources. *Meat, cheese, butter, milk and eggs* are sources of animal fats. Certain fats cannot be made by the body yet are essential to cell health, so a tablespoon of fat or oil per day is necessary; Westerners generally consume six times that amount. The liver breaks fats down into glycerol (for cell energy) and fatty acids (used in the metabolic process). As you are probably well aware, excess fat in the diet is stored as body fat!

4 **Wonderful water**: essential to life; 60 per cent of your body mass is water. It's in blood, in the tissue fluids that nurture cells, in every cell. It maintains body temperature, aids digestion, dilutes waste products and helps their elimination. You excrete about 2 litres (about 4 pints) of water per day. Most foods contain a lot of water (fruit and vegetables, for instance), but an additional 1.5 litres (3 pints) of fluids daily is necessary.

5 **Feelgood fibre**: required by the body for the elimination phase of food digestion. Fibre, also called roughage, is the indigestible part of food called cellulose, found in *vegetables, fruits and wholegrains*. Muscles move waste matter along the bowel, but this movement occurs only when the intestinal walls are stretched sufficiently by the bulk of the waste matter. Too little bulk (fibre) leads to sluggish movement and constipation, delaying elimination of waste. This can leave you feeling heavy and low, and can result in poor skin.

6 & 7 **Sparky minerals and vitamins**: vital to the body's ability to use nutrients, as spark plugs are to igniting fuel in a car engine. Some minerals and vitamins have particular jobs to do (such as skin cell growth or movement of oxygen), some are essential for all metabolism. Minerals are inorganic and are sometimes called mineral salts. The body contains a great deal of some minerals (calcium in bones, potassium in cells, for example). It has a need for eight major minerals and about six trace elements. Vitamins are organic and, though not part of body structure like many of the minerals, they are necessary for metabolism. Some vitamins are carried and stored via fats, others are carried only by water, which means they cannot be stored in the body. Fortunately, all the minerals and vitamins essential to life are found in foods normally included in a healthy diet, such as *eggs, milk, cheese,*

green vegetables, fish, meat. If you are thinking of taking supplements, note these points:
- Minerals and vitamins are useless on their own; take them with a meal.
- Minerals equal vitamins in importance, and vice versa.
- RDA on the label means Recommended Daily Allowance, the minimum required to prevent deficiency disease.
- Food quality, lifestyle (caffeine intake, smoking, alcohol intake, medication, pollution, stress), and eating habits interfere with vitamin/mineral intake and uptake; nutritionists recommend an intake higher than the RDA for special needs and optimum health.
- If you want to take booster doses of minerals or vitamins you should take multi-minerals/vitamins because they all interact and depend on each other to work.
- Excess amounts of some minerals and vitamins are toxic; check with a doctor, qualified complementary medicine practitioner or specialist self-help book before embarking on a supplement programme.

Vital vitamins and minerals

Vitamin/mineral	Helps
A	Many eye problems, immune system, hair, skin.
B complex	Nerves, depression, irritability, mental alertness, fatigue, breast milk, PMS, alcoholism, skin, greying hair, Alzheimer's disease.
C	Healing, colds, stress, viruses, cholesterol, allergies, skin, bleeding gums.
D	Absorption of calcium for bone strength.
E	Tiredness, bloating, ageing, healing, fertility.
Calcium	Strong bones, teeth, heart, insomnia, period cramps.
Iron	Disease resistance, fatigue, anaemia, skin tone.
Magnesium	Depression, vertigo, PMS, cramps, morning sickness, alcoholism.
Zinc	Eczema, hair loss, healing, fertility, mental alertness, cholesterol, irregular periods.
Iodine	Thyroid gland, metabolism.
Phosphorus	Teeth, bones, function of B vitamins.

Ease into better eating

How can you switch to a healthier eating style? You have to find what works for you. Maybe you want a real regime – magazines and books offer a host of diets you can try, or you can join a Weight Watchers group. Perhaps you don't want to embark on a major change in your eating habits, but you would like to improve your diet. But maybe you have already been down these routes and failed. The trouble is that the novelty and motivation of a special diet wear off. You get bored or it's too finicky or you need a treat – and all the good is undone.

> Here's a way to sneak up on yourself and ease into better eating patterns. First, always, before any new diet or exercise programme, check with your doctor. This will ensure you are basically fit and ready to get pro-actively fit: your doctor is sure to approve.

Ease-in plan: drink more

Start simply by drinking that 1.5 litres (3 pints) of fluid we should all drink daily – only make it just water. Treat yourself to a big bottle of non-fizzy spring water, or just fill up a 2-litre bottle or a measured jug. Keep it on your desk, or in your kitchen, or wherever you spend most of your time, and sip away the whole bottle during the course of your day. You can have fruit juices, soft drinks or coffee or tea as well, if you wish, but after a few water-added days, give up the caffeinated drinks. This isn't a permanent sacrifice, just a two- or three- week caffeine break to clear out your system. Caffeine is a stimulant, a toxin, a drug. If you feel irritable, and perhaps have a nagging little headache for two or three days, that usually means you have had a caffeine addiction. Caffeine detracts from a normal, healthy balanced state. A hot beverage is soothing, it's true, and it can substitute for snacking, so go ahead and have one, but make it

- hot water with a squeeze or slice of lemon (this aids digestion, especially first thing in the morning)
- a herbal tea
- hot chocolate for a now-and-then treat
- South American matte herbal tea (this is bitter but mildly caffeinated; try it if you just can't do without a fix).

FUELLING YOUR POWERHOUSE: HEALTHY EATING

Ease-in plan: eat more

Begin to increase the amount of fresh fruit and vegetables you eat. Have a whole orange or half a grapefruit with breakfast, an apple with lunch, a salad with dinner (plus your usual cooked vegetables). Between meals, if you feel hungry, drink water and/or eat another apple, pear, orange, satsuma, small bunch of grapes. If this sounds too drastic, go on, have a snack biscuit, but eat the piece of fruit (or cut up carrot, celery, cucumber or other raw vegetable) before you eat the sweet thing.

Begin to increase the complex carbohydrates you eat, such as wholemeal breads, cereals, pasta. Think brown whenever possible and reduce the white, refined versions of the same foods. In place of meat and poultry (which can provide protein-and-fat-overload) as main dishes: have more jacket potatoes with butter/margarine and cheese, cottage cheese, fish grilled, baked or poached, stir-fries with brown rice, pasta (avoid creamy sauces).

Increase your use of spices and herbs to make lower-fat foods and smaller portions satisfyingly tasty. They aid digestion, too. Try foreign cuisines: Chinese, Indian, Thai and others are often high on taste and healthiness.

Nutrition tricks and timing

Tips: sugar high, sugar low, sugar secrets

Scientific experiments indicate that sugar doesn't satisfy hunger; it actually creates it. Hunger occurs when blood sugar levels fall. When you eat a meal or snack, sugars in food stimulate insulin production, and the insulin removes excess sugar from the blood and stores it in the liver or as fat. In most people a chunk of sugar, like a chocolate bar, triggers a surge of insulin which works extra efficiently to mop up the excess sugar. Within an hour there may be less sugar in the blood than there was before the sugary snack. This low blood sugar level may lead to lethargy and a hunger for another sweet bite – and so the cycle goes on, fuelled by the body's own balancing system. Remove sugars from the cycle and you solve the problem. If you substitute slow-release carbohydrates (such as wholemeal bread) or high fibre, mineral and vitamin sugar-bearers (apples, grapes, etc.) the blood sugar doesn't surge so dramatically, so you feel satisfied for longer.

- Swap six teaspoons of sugar a day for two apples and a banana. Same calories, better nutrition.
- Sugar causes tooth decay. Saliva clears out the mouth in an hour or so. So whatever you do, don't have a sweet snack every hour or you'll rot your teeth *and* get fat.
- Honey and brown sugar are nutritionally no better than white sugar.
- Hidden sugar: manufactured savoury snacks such as crisps often contain sugar, salt and fats – humans' natural baby-taste pleasers.
- Use sugar substitute sweeteners, low-calorie drinks to gradually wean yourself off sugar and sugary foods towards cleaner, non-sweet tastes.

Tips: fat good, fat bad, fat tricks

A little bit of fat is good for you, but it has to be the right kind. Fats, oils, lipids – biochemically they're all in one general category. 'Bad' fats, called saturated fats, are mostly found in animal fats and are solid at room temperature (butter, double cream, fat on meat). Solid outside, solid inside: they turn to dense blood fats, cholesterol, and fur up arteries, paving the way for heart attacks and strokes. These 'bad' fats are also thought to lead to breast cancer in some women.

'Good' fats, called unsaturated fats, are mostly found in plants (and some fish) and are liquid at room temperature. Broken down by the body into unsaturated fatty acids, some of these are vital to life: so vital that they are called essential fatty acids, EFAs. They are elemental in cell walls (see Chapter 1), hormones, and skin moisture retention. They even help reduce the risk of heart disease.

Also on the healthy side, unsaturated fats contain vitamins A, D, E, K, important to skin, bones and fertility. A bit of fat or oil has great digestive advantages, too: it slows down the rate at which food gets from the stomach to the small intestines, so you feel satisfied longer.

- To keep hunger at bay, try some avocado in your salad, a scrape of butter on your wholemeal bread, a teaspoon of olive oil on your pasta or some cheese on your jacket potato.
- Take skin off chicken and turkey after cooking to halve their fat content.

- Semi-skimmed milk has only 2 per cent fat, skimmed milk 1 per cent, far less than normal milk. Acquire the taste.
- Cut down on supersaturated fat foods – sausages, hard cheeses, salami, cream, butter, fat-edged and fat-marbled meats, eggs.
- Switch to unsaturated sunflower, safflower or cold-pressed virgin olive oil. Increase unsaturated oily fish such as herring, sardines, tuna, salmon.

Tips: why raw, why wholemeal?

Thousands of years ago, humans invented cooking to make meat and other foods digestible. Today's way often takes all the 'undigestibles' out of food and the result is white flour, white rice, ground-up, air-puffed cereals, snacks and biscuits. Unnecessary sugar and salt are usually added to this highly refined food which is, in effect, predigested; essential natural nutrients such as fibre, minerals and vitamins have been removed. Fibre is the structure and skin of plant foods and is at its best when raw or minimally processed. You need it for healthy elimination (see Chapter 1). Minerals and vitamins are concentrated just below the skin of fruit and vegetables; if you eat these foods unpeeled and raw or only lightly cooked the nutrients won't be scraped away or leached into cooking water.

- Eat more foods such as fresh apples, raw celery, uncooked mushrooms, beansprout salad, potatoes cooked and eaten with the skin on, muesli full of rolled oats, nuts and raisins, wholemeal or wholewheat bread. Green peas, by the way, are among the highest-fibre vegetables because of the skin around each little pea.
- When you cook vegetables, cook them quickly and lightly in a small amount of water, or steam them, or stir fry. The aim is to have them fresh-coloured, still crunchy, not soggy and bland.
- Start and/or end every meal with raw fruit or vegetables for two good reasons. The natural sugars and crunchiness get digestive juices flowing fast, for efficient food processing. And your taste buds get educated towards clean, healthy foods, away from pure sugary, stodgy, salty or fatty foods. Start a meal with crudités, salad or simply a nibble of celery to cleanse your palate and set you up to eat and digest well. At the end, fresh fruit salad gives you a sweet, clean, refreshing conclusion. Try it a few times instead of double chocolate fudge cake or cheesecake – you'll begin to prefer fruit.

Tips: happy-hour ambush – salt and alcohol

An average Western diet includes two teaspoonfuls (12 g/ $^1/_2$ oz) of salt daily, which is about ten times more than necessary. In fact if you added no salt to your food at table or in cooking and you managed to eat no processed food with salt, you'd still get double your needs from the salt that's naturally in foods. High salt intake is implicated in high blood pressure which strains the heart and increases the risk of heart attack and strokes. Highly salted food is a taste we learn to like, and it's often combined with fat and sugar in calorific crisps, salted nuts and other cocktail snacks – it whets the appetite for more of the same, and creates thirst, too. It's just too bad if the liquid to hand is alcoholic, because beer, wine and spirits are loaded with calories – 50 in a standard measure of vodka (about as low as you can go, not counting the mixer), 75 or more in a glass of wine. What's more, alcohol provides virtually no nutrients and is a burden on the liver, which has to burn it up and get it out of your system. A unit of alcohol (a small glass of wine, a single measure of spirit or a half-pint of beer) or even two units a day is reasonable and may even do you good, but more than this is asking for trouble.

- Retrain your palate by reducing salt intake; natural flavours are tasty if you let them be so.
- Salt substitutes are expensive – use them to wean you off salt, but only for a while.
- Drink a glass of water for every glass of alchohol, alternating throughout the evening.
- Dilute your drink with a mixer; sip slowly; top up with pure mixer.
- Give your liver a rest by having two or three alcohol-free days per week.
- Substitute cut-up raw vegetables and a dip for salty snacks, have tomato or other fruit juice, or mineral waters instead of alcohol.

Tips: emotional food factors

Food is a comfort, a reward, a revenge, a treat, a habit. Note how often, when and what you eat; ask yourself what drives you to eat. Is it genuine body hunger, stomach pangs or rumbles? Is it a normal meal time? Between meals, or after a meal but before having a second helping or desert, think – are you really hungry? Or are you anxious, depressed, angry, sad, bored, or simply doing what you always do? Sometimes an emotional need overwhelms your body's own real desires for wholesome, clean food. Emotions can also cause you not to eat. This is natural enough when you grieve, but not good if you're tense about work or relationships, or suffering the self-loathing of an anorexic or bulimic eater.

Escape the emotional food factor by tuning into your feelings before, during and after your meals and snacks. Try substituting healthier food. Decide if this hunger really needs to be fed this way right now. As you eat more healthy, sustaining foods and eat regular balanced meals, work towards reducing your comfort treat habits. Increase fresh fruit as snacks and desserts, try to get down to one treat a day, maybe only two or three a week?

Tips: when is a diet not a diet?

When and how you eat is part of the healthy good-looks pattern. Have three meals a day and don't skip any. People who do tend to reward their 'goodness' or refuel themselves by over-indulging at the next meal.

Breakfast builds performance: after the fast of a night's sleep, you need to refuel your system. Porridge or muesli is ideal because oats are digested slowly and milk provides a bit of natural sugar and fat, all totalling hunger satisfaction. Sprinkle on raisins, sunflower seeds or nuts, if you like, for bonus vitamins, minerals, fibre and EFAs. Add a piece of fresh fruit and some herbal tea, and you're launched.

If you are of the just-a-coffee-and-piece-of-toast habit, try out the above healthy breakfast regime for two weeks. Toast or a bun alone provides less fibre than muesli and releases its energy more quickly, the coffee boosts you up, then drops you – you feel hungry sooner.

Lunch around midday comes just before the natural human downtime of mid-afternoon. The body is made to have lunch, so give it what it needs. Try to take a break from whatever you are doing, sit down to eat in a calm and orderly way. This aids digestion and eases tensions.

Dinner, like lunch, a balanced meal of healthy foods, should be relaxing and pleasurable. If you've eaten correctly all day you won't feel the need to eat extra or extra-rich food. Some experts believe that a high-protein meal fuels you for a high performance event the next day, while a high-carbohydrate meal provides for solid, steady performance. So you might want to try grilled steak, chicken or fish the night before your big presentation, interview or tennis match, and have pasta the night following to help you wind down.

Predictable patterns of progress (or not)

As you follow the 'Eat more', 'Drink more' guides and the know-how 'Tips' you'll educate your taste buds and tune in to your body for better head-to-toe beauty. But anticipate the following resistance:

- **First three days** – Resolve and sense of adventure at first. Then feeling of deprivation, difficulty, impossibility. Perhaps headache, fatigue as your body does without caffeine.
- **Week 1** – Frustration, boredom, annoyance, doubt. Will this really work? Why bother? You can drink less water now, if you wish, but try to keep up a reasonable intake.
- **Week 2** – Annoyance, resentment continue, but you're getting used to doing without caffeine and regular sugar/salt snacks, even though you still very much want them.
- **Week 3** – Still wanting usual snack/sweet habits, and by now you've slipped and had some, but apples, salads and lightly cooked vegetables have become user-friendly. Good taste habits are setting in.
- **Week 4** – Permission to try coffee, tea, a biscuit, sugary snack. Strangely, they may not taste as good as you thought they would. This means you have broken the habit. Try to continue on this 'deprived' level, but you can now have caffeine, snacks, puddings occasionally when you want them, but only when you really do want them. Keep up the healthy eating evolution.
- **Month 2** – Keep adding the good stuff: wholemeal, raw fruit/vegetables. Also, keep deleting the not-so-good: fatty meats and dairy products, sugary and salty things. This way of life is becoming less of a novelty now, though still a challenge.
- **Month 3** – Clean, healthy eating patterns are well established, with the freedom to have a treat now and then – but without caffeine or sweetness as a regular habit.
- **Tuned in** – As you gear up to healthier eating patterns you may or may not lose weight and change body shape, but for sure your skin, nails, hair and general sparkle will be better. Over the two or three months of evolving, your general health should improve, you'll have more energy, enthusiasm and optimism. Success builds success, so as you get used to your new eating style you may be motivated to go on a stricter portion-controlled or calorie-counting diet if you need to lose further weight.

But the main point of this simple detoxifying healthy eating style is to encourage you to listen to your body in order to gain good looks. Tune in to what it wants – clean, crunchy, wholesome tastes and sensations – not what you give it unthinkingly, not what it wants out of habit.

SNACKS, TREATS AND SINS (AND FORGIVENESS)

Snacks are okay, if you need them, if they're constructive. You want to avoid the sugar-hunger rebound cycle, so avoid biscuits and chocolate bars. Instead, when you feel hungry between meals try

- an apple
- any other kind of raw fruit or vegetables
- herbal tea
- sunflower seeds or unsalted nuts
- a glass of semi-skimmed milk
- a few raisins
- a muesli bar.

The last two are rather high in calories, and the milk is more like a meal because of its protein content, but at least these are all healthy, nutritional foods, not empty, pure-fatty calories.

Don't be a saint. This is a long-term eating pattern you're working on, not a sprint. You want to retune your taste buds gradually, so if you can't resist that banoffee pie when you're out, then have it (maybe halve it and share it with a companion?). Just keep up your water intake, your fresh fruit and vegetables, the regular balanced meals.

If (when) you fall back into old ways, don't punish yourself. You have started, you have made progress. It is human to relapse. It's not the end of the world and not a reason to give up your determination to look good and be healthy. Forgive yourself, go to your favourite greengrocer and treat yourself to the juiciest apples, freshest watercress, brightest oranges, crispest beansprouts and the current seasonal fruit. Take your cornucopia home and make a meal of encouragement.

3
ENERGISING YOUR POWERHOUSE: EXERCISE

The best reason for exercise is to pump oxygen and healthy nutrients through your system to nurture every cell and to carry away the wastes of cell life processes. Exercise also brings large-scale good looks, good life benefits: action, strength, flexibility, skin and muscle tone, body shape, mental alertness.

If you already have a favourite sport, say tennis or skiing, you know that you enjoy using your body actively and keeping it in shape so that you play well and safely. Swimming, of course, is an excellent all-over exercise. If you exercise regularly, congratulations, keep it up. If you do little or nothing, and wish you could keep it that way, read on.

Ease into exercise

Even if a beautiful new you is your only goal, any new bodystyle pattern you try (eating or exercise) is bound to flop if you go at it with grim determination. The obstacles and excuses are endless: I'm too busy, I hate exercising, I'm too old, I'm too tired, I'm not fit, I'm fit enough already....

To make exercise a habit you enjoy, you need to operate by the pleasure principle. What do you like? What will fit into your life? By finding the right exercise for you and your life demands, you can evolve into a healthier new bodystyle. So if you are naturally orderly, sociable, fashion conscious or poorly disciplined try exercise via the routine and people-interaction of a gym or a class. Competitive, sociable people tend to like sports. Nature lovers, the budget-conscious and solitude lovers should try walking, running, cycling. Sensualists want a gym or club with a sauna and whirlpool. Shy or time-pressed people will be happier with workout videos and equipment to use at home, or a personal trainer, if budget allows. Know yourself, be realistic and creatively flexible about getting exercise into your life.

> ### CHECK BEFORE YOU START
> As with new eating styles, see your doctor before embarking on a new exercise programme to be sure blood pressure, lungs and heart are in basic good working order.

Ease-in plan: toe first

As with eating patterns, you should ease exercise into your life gradually. Start by just putting your toe into the exercise water, say, with morning or lunchtime stretches. After one week, add to one day a 20 to 30-minute aerobic/toning session (including warm up/down). Add a second of these sessions to another day in the second week. Add additional walks. You'll begin to tune in to your body. After three weeks or so you may be surprised to feel that your body calls for more. Gradually add more exercise, increasing your staying power: a third session a week, more stretches, two extra lengths of the pool, five minutes more of dancing, a half-mile longer or uphill walk/run/cycle. Do it – enjoy it!

After four to six weeks you'll feel stale, sluggish, restless if you skip exercising. Good, you're starting to establish the exercise habit.

It takes at least 20 minutes of continuous hard-breathing exercise three times a week to be fully fit. To lose weight, increase this to four or five times a week. You also need muscle-specific exercise for toning, strength, suppleness. (Details follow later in this chapter.)

Something is better than nothing. If you simply can't or won't do the ideal, don't give up. Do just a little; do what you can.

How muscles work

It will help your exercise willpower and enjoyment, and your good-looks goals, to know just how exercise works. Your body has thousands of muscles. Involuntary muscles (heartbeat, intestinal movement of food bulk, etc.) aren't usually under your control, though emotions can affect them. Voluntary muscles (reaching, running, kicking, carrying, bending) are the ones you can exercise to increase strength, stamina and suppleness. Included here is the sheath of muscles under your skin that accounts for skin's firmness and contour.

Muscle fibres, which make up the whole muscle, can stretch and return to their original size and shape: they are elastic. Skin and a layer of fat cover your muscles; supple and protective, they move when muscles move. For most movements one major muscle contracts and a corresponding one relaxes. Try it: bend your arm at the elbow and feel the biceps in the upper arm tauten, feel the triceps under the upper arm – it's slack.

Muscles can lose elasticity in a number of ways. They can be flabby from under-use (have you ever seen how a limb looks after it's been in a plaster cast for weeks?), or from over-use (creases from nose to mouth as you age). Muscles and skin are subject to gravity, which can eventually make them sag. Muscles, and the tendons and ligaments that attach them to bones, can be torn or overstretched by too violent or vigorous movement. Being living tissue, muscle can usually repair itself, and this is the basis of exercise. Careful, planned, gentle damage, achieved through repeated, gradually increased muscle movement, causes muscles to gain in strength and elasticity. The result is that even at rest a well-toned muscle is firm, not flabby. The trick of good exercise is to contract and relax your various muscles in various directions to strengthen (tone) all their fibres.

Warm-up, warm-down, why?

For any of the exercise groups that follow, even if you are super fit, you must get supple to prevent muscle injury. Warming up or down feels good, like a luxurious cat stretch, with added gentle side bends, toe touches, calf stretches, waist twists, head rotations, arm swings and simple pacing about (see 'Get stretched' on page 32).

Muscles can tear with sudden effort. Warm-ups let fibres gently stretch, start blood flowing, ready for action.

When warming down, afterwards, be sure to release or relax the muscles you've been working on, which means contracting each muscle's opposite partner. Following the biceps tautening example above, relax the biceps by reaching overhead and trying to touch the back of your shoulder – you can feel that the triceps is stretched, the biceps loose.

Warm-down has another advantage: working muscles create lactic acid, a waste product which the speeded-up blood circulation carries away. If you stop suddenly, circulation slows rapidly and some waste remains, resulting in sore muscles.

Stop exercising

Yes: muscles build strength by repairing and recovering from vigorous work, so they need a break. Do aerobics only on alternate days. You can intersperse with muscle toning/strengthening, or else be sure to exercise different muscle groups in a cycle of days. It's fine to do stretching and breathing work every day.

Seven exercise routes

1 Get puffed

If you can do only one kind of exercise, do something aerobic. This is exercise that gets you a bit breathless and keeps you moving your arms and legs rhythmically. 'Aerobic' stems from the word air – you take oxygen from the air to release energy. Aerobic exercise helps stamina and general muscle tone but most of all it works heart and lungs, the internal health system that leads to better energy and better-looking skin and hair.

You need to do it for 20 to 30 minutes three times a week, and it can be as easy as a brisk walk or as sophisticated as a gym workout. Other examples include: swimming, jogging (running), bicycling, dancing, skipping with a rope, stair climbing, trampolining, home video workouts, home cycling or rowing. It should involve your whole body in rhythmic, repetitive, continuous movement, so that you breathe hard after a few minutes at it and you begin to glow or even sweat with perspiration. Though breathing heavily, you should be able to talk or sing during and after the exercise – not gasp and collapse on the floor.

Don't leap into this suddenly. Follow the warm-up/down section techniques, and ease gradually into this new regime. Walk, climb stairs, swim or whatever for three minutes, rest, then another three minutes, repeat. Or set distances as goals. After a week or two your body will actually want to work longer between rests. If you attend a class or gym, be sure the instructor knows you are starting from zero and you need a gradual build-up. Don't rush it: you will injure muscles and undermine motivation. In 6 weeks you'll be able to keep up 20 minutes of non-stop aerobics, and you'll be proud of yourself, feel more alive and in possession of a different body.

For running or vigorous workouts wear running shoes to absorb the shock of pounding feet as they hit the ground. Be pleased that any of the foot-pounding exercises help build strong bones, vital for women because bones get weaker after the menopause. Be sure to wear a bra to support breast tissue.

2 Get toned

To firm specific areas of your body, like flabby upper arms, soft tummy, wobbly thighs, love handles (I could go on) you need to concentrate on local muscle groups with anaerobic exercise. This means you contract your muscles to make them work, but you do not necessarily get out of breath. Keep-fit classes and gym and home workouts and home videos provide these exercises. Many are simple and basic, a few might be better to learn under supervision, to be sure you get them right. As with aerobics, warm up/down and work at a tortoise pace at first: 3 repetitions of each, then 5, then 10, up to 30 as your muscle strength grows.

You can do these tone-anaerobics for a 20-minute session up to 3 days a week, alternating with your hard breathing aerobic days. Or you can alternate aerobic and toning exercises in a single longer session, using the toners as a break from the puffers.

ENERGISING YOUR POWERHOUSE: EXERCISE

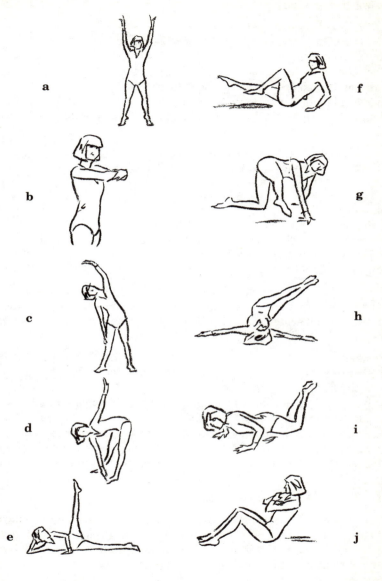

Figure 2 Get toned

What tones what?

Standing-up exercises
Sky reach for arms, waist – see illustration 2a
Arm circles for arms, bust
Bust jumper for arms, bust – see illustration 2b
Side bend reach for waist, hip – see illustration 2c
Side bend no-hands for waist, midriff
Windmill reach for waist, lower back, thighs – see illustration 2d

Floorwork
Side leg lifts for thighs, hips, waist – see illustration 2e
Sit kicks for abdomen, thighs – see illustration 2f
Leg stirs for thighs, waist, bottom – see illustration 2g
Legs tick tock for abdomen, lower back, waist, hips, midriff – see illustration 2h
Half push-ups for arms, bust – see illustration 2i
Semi sit-ups for abdomen – see illustration 2j, but arms straight
Roll-ups for abdomen – see illustration 2j
Knee squeeze for bottom, thighs, hips – see illustration 3d

Some of these will be more difficult for you than others, depending on your muscle strength. You may feel a little muscle soreness (not strain) the following day, which is fine. It'll go as you continue to use muscles.

Remember:
- Do **not** hold your breath as you contract or stretch. Breathe out with effort, it aids the exercise.
- If anything gives you pain, stop. Do it only half-way; gradually the pain barrier will recede.
- Breasts do not have muscles, but they are supported by muscles. Though exercise cannot reduce or enlarge breasts, stronger support muscles can improve the line of your bust and help posture.

3 Get stretched

You need another specific element for real fitness: flexibility. These exercises are gentle, slow stretches to create supple muscles and joints. Easy and relaxing, they are an aid to better posture, which is crucial to beauty and personal style (see Chapter 6). They're also an excellent antidote to stress (more on stress in Chapter 10).

ENERGISING YOUR POWER

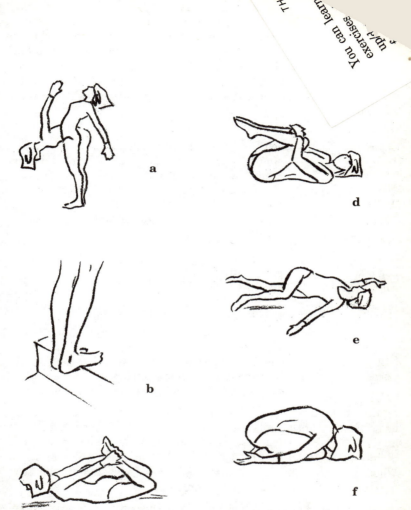

Figure 3 Get stretched

ese in a yoga class, and many are used in toning
ordinary keep-fit classes and in aerobic warming
 .n. You use your mind, not brute energy, to gain flexibility,
 eeling the stretch, becoming aware of tension, letting it go. The main
aim is to stretch into a position, and then relax into it further and let
the stretch gently go further, staying in the position for three or four
complete breaths. Always remember to breathe throughout each exercise – holding the breath creates muscle tension, the opposite of what
you want.

Standing

Sky reach	– see 'Get Toned', illustration 2a
Toe touch	– simply bend over at waist and let head and arms hang down, or gently stretch arms towards toes
Chest expansion	– see illustration 3a
Waist circle	– hands on hips, hold lower body still and make wide circles from the waist with the upper body
Calf stretch	– see illustration 3b

Floorwork

Leg bow	– see illustration 3c
Knee hold	– see illustration 3d
Knee roll	– see illustration 3e
Legover	– this is the same as knee roll, but extend (don't bend) the crossover leg, and extend both arms on the floor at shoulder level
Egg	– see illustration 3f
Corpse	– basic warm-down for stretches: lie on back, arms at side, release body, feel heavy on the floor

Another easy fixer is to roll a small face towel into a firm cylinder and lie on the floor with it aligned lengthwise along your upper spine. You may need a book under the back of your head to prevent neck strain. Simply lie there on the towel and breathe for three to five minutes. When you rise, you'll find that your chest feels more open, you breathe better, neck and shoulders are less tense.

As you can see (and feel!) these exercises concentrate on lengthening and stretching you to counteract physical tensions, body misuse and gravity.

Do these first thing in the morning or last thing at night, in a lunch break or coffee break, or integrate them with toners or aerobic warm-up/down.

4 Get strong

Actual muscle strength – how much weight a muscle group can lift or pull, and for how long or how often — grows through both aerobic and anaerobic toning exercises. Strong muscles keep their tone even at rest, so these exercises are good for firming thighs, buttocks, upper arm, abdomen. Weight work builds up bone strength, too, important from age 40 onwards. To build strength use gym machines (with professional advice) or barbells (graduated weights), or weighted wrist/ankle bands. You can also simply fill plastic bottles with water; grasp them as you perform arm lifts, gradually increasing the amount of water as you gain strength. Use these home-made barbells with any of the arm exercises listed under 'What tones what?' on page 32. Build up gradually in a 6 to 8 to 12-week programme, combining with aerobics, stretch and tone routines. You'll see a tautness, feel firmness in arm/leg muscles. Don't worry about getting gleaming muscle bulges; women's muscles are smoother than men's and it would take super-dedicated effort to get a pumping-iron look to your biceps.

5 Get a lungful

As well as hard-breathing aerobic exercise, simple, conscious deep breathing can increase your oxygenation easily and give great benefits to lungs, mental and physical vitality, and to hair, nails and complexion.

Try the Complete Yoga Breath – mentally count nine as you slowly breathe in through your nose, pushing out your abdomen first, then your entire chest. Hold for a moment, then slowly exhale through your nose to a mental count of nine. Repeat three times. You can do this standing, sitting or lying down. If desired, you can slowly raise your arms to overhead with the first count of nine, and lower them as you breathe out. Gradually build up to ten repetitions.

Sing, join a choir, do dramatics, take voice classes, learn to play a recorder, flute or other wind instrument – besides being fun and creative, activities like these, along with aerobics and conscious deep breathing, exercise your lungs and improve body oxygenation. The availability of oxygen and release of carbon dioxide feeds brain, skin, all aspects of being.

6 Stop puffing

Give up smoking – what? That's not exercise! Technically, no, but smoking so interferes with your body that breaking the cigarette habit is a route to good looks all on its own. Smoking clogs up your lungs, blocking oxygen absorption and permanently damaging them. It causes heart disease, lung cancer, emphysyma, other lung diseases. It enlarges your pores. It leathers your skin. It makes your hands, hair, clothes and breath smell. It destroys your vitamin C intake. If you smoke to feel cool, grown-up and sophisticated, think how much more cool and in control you'll feel having beaten the demon. If you smoke to relax and relieve tension out of habit, substitute the Complete Yoga Breath and aerobic exercise; sip away at your 1.5 litres of water, eat apples.

It's not easy, but you can do it. There are lots of ways to break the habit. Your GP, self-help books or organisations (see addresses at the back of this book) will guide you through. The main secret is to be motivated. If you do care about beauty and health – well, you know smoking destroys both.

7 Get sexy

Exercise your sex muscle – you can do it any time, anywhere, it's sexy to do and it's good for sex. Even more important, it helps prevent incontinence in your later years – the embarrassing, uncontrolled leaking of urine. After childbirth, women are advised by a physiotherapist to do this to help recovery of the vaginal muscle tone. But you can and should start at any age. Simply clench your vaginal sphinctre muscle and hold the contraction for a count of three. Think of it as trying to keep a tampon from falling out. Release and repeat four times. Gradually build up the length of time you can hold each clench; aim for an eventual ten seconds. Notice how buttocks and urethral (urine outlet) muscles contract, too – the whole region gets toned. Remember to breathe as you do this; it takes some mental concentration at first.

Make love – a satisfying lovemaking session is great for beauty and health. Your heart beats faster, circulation speeds up, blood diffuses to the surface of your skin so it flushes and softens, you perspire slightly – all great for complexion and microcirculation. Plus, if you are a female in bed with a male, there's a good chance your complexion will get a lovely exfoliating scruffing from his whiskers.

Of course, it'll help you get to the lovemaking stage if you have healthy good looks to start with ....

POWERHOUSE RALLY

I repeat, it's not instant and it's not a pushover to train yourself to new, healthy, beauty eating and exercise patterns. That's why you should ease into new ways. Some tips:

- If you try and fail, or don't try at all, ask yourself: Are you afraid of change? Fearful that a better looking you would have to fight off admirers? Do you secretly condemn pretty people as arrogant? Feel safer hiding under extra flesh? Don't let a hidden agenda undermine you; air it and conquer it. Consider counselling, if necessary. You have a right to be proud of yourself and your looks.
- Keep a diary or notebook of your decisions, actions, a record of your small achievements, failures. It helps you feel responsible for your beauty ambition and progress.
- Reward yourself for sticking with it. Ideally not with food. Perhaps a haircut or manicure (see Chapter 9), a pair of earrings or wild socks, a book or magazine, fragrance, a lipstick...
- Settle for less. If you keep trying and failing, lower your sights. There must be something you can do.
- Cut out motivating magazine pictures, headlines, postcards to remind you, inspire you, make you laugh. Stick them on your fridge, kitchen cupboards, bedroom/bathroom mirror, desk.
- Talk about it. Make new acquaintances at gym, pool, class. Share routines, ideas, successes, moans.
- Don't talk about it. Family and friends tend to tease. Just ease into new ways; don't state big intentions. And don't be a health, beauty and style bore — life and you are more interesting than calories, clothes and looks.
- If you feel too tired, depressed, stressed out or busy, remember that exercise gives you more energy, not less. It also reduces stress and depression, making you feel in control of your time. At least go for a long, hard walk.
- Accept failures. They will happen. Don't stop. Evolve. Keep going in your small (triumphant) way. Grow gradually to establish new habits, new health, great new looks.

4

PUTTING YOUR BEST FACE FORWARD: SKIN

Now is the time to focus on the skin-deep aspects of looking good, starting with skin itself, because clear, soft skin is the essence of good looks.

Two-part self-assessment: what's your skin type?

Part 1

You are one of four main ethnic skin types; each has advantages and disadvantages.

Type/description	Advantages	Disadvantages
Caucasian (white). Pale beige, possibly with pink or yellow tones.	Can be translucent and fine-pored.	Can be delicate, show age early. Risk of sunburn, skin cancer.
Oriental, fair Asian. Creamy ivory, possibly yellow or olive tones.	Rarely has pimples, blackheads or shows age.	Scars easily; sometimes uneven pigmentation.
Mediterranean, Latina, dark Asian. Brownish melanin pigmentation with yellow-red tone.	Not difficult; tans easily; ages late.	May be oily; possible excess hair.
African, Afro-Caribbean (black). Melanin pigments, skin medium to very deep brown, sometimes with blue, red or yellow tones.	Smooth, supple; ages very late.	May be shiny. Rapid cell-shedding. Scars easily.

Part 2

You are also one of four main sebacious types. Sebum is the oil your skin naturally produces to protect itself.

Type/description	Problems	Advantages
Balanced. Soft and supple because an even balance of sebum and moisture emerges from skin's deeper layers.	None. Small pores, healthy colour, smooth and clear: all because of good micro-circulation and because cell shedding and growth occur at same rate. Rare pimples, blackheads heal easily.	This is the ideal!
Dry. Dull uneven texture, lacks suppleness, may feel tight; pores invisible, skin thin; fine lines and wrinkles before other skin types: all because there is insufficient sebum.	Cheeks and nose may be pink or red: capillaries dilated, skin unable to protect itself.	In youth you may be an 'English rose'.
Oily. Shiny, coarse, dull, due to sebum overproduction. Grimy grey-yellow, thick: sebum layer slows cells shedding, they build up unevenly.	Pores large, maybe blackheads, pimples: excess sebum stretches and blocks pores.	Your skin looks younger longer.
Combination. Characteristics of balanced, dry, or oily skin in various places on the face: uneven sebum production.	T-zone is the most typical pattern: oily forehead, nose and chin with balanced or dry cheeks, eye area.	You get the good (but also, alas, the bad) points of the other skin types.

You may also be one or more of four challenged skin types: sensitive, dehydrated, troubled, ageing/mature. Their details and management are covered later in this chapter.

THE HEALTH AND BEAUTY HANDBOOK

Skin know-how

So now you know your skin type – how to preserve its good points and counteract its problems? If you know how skin works you'll know what to do and why to do it.

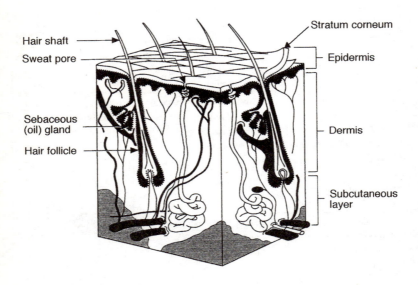

Figure 4 Skin deep: a cross-section

Your skin is a major organ of protection, a sensual communicator, a vital conveyor of waste, a temperature regulator. It covers your entire body, and its upper layer, the epidermis, which we generally think of as skin, is only 1 mm thick at its thickest (the palms and soles).

Your skin is constantly renewing itself, a living miracle of self-replacement. Deep epidermal cells push up to the outer layer and become hard protein cells bound on to the top surface. These top cells, the skin you see and touch, are actually dead, but they are supple and form the tight barrier that keeps germs out and moisture in. This is the *stratum corneum* layer of the epidermis.

It takes about six months for a new skin cell to mature at the bottom layer of the epidermis, and a further two weeks to push its way to the top where it stays for another two weeks before being shed. With this timescale you can see how a new regime of healthy eating and exercise will take time to show its benefits – but it will show. Skin cell regeneration generally happens when you're asleep, from midnight to 4 a.m., while body metabolism is slow, saving energy for the work of making skin.

Below the epidermis is a deeper layer of skin called the dermis which contains blood capillaries and lymph which deliver nutrients to and remove wastes from the lowest epidermal layer which generates the new cells (see 'Cell power', Chapter 1, and 'Beating illness', Chapter 10). When you cut yourself and bleed, you've reached the dermis. It also contains various nerve endings (pain, heat, cold, pressure) that transmit sensation. Lower down in the dermis is a layer dense with renewing connective protein fibres: collagen for flexible strength, elastin able to stretch and return to its original shape, and reticulin to hold it all in place.

Finally, the subcutaneous layer contains fatty tissue to insulate and cushion the body. It also 'plumps out' the skin providing contours – think of a baby's face. Rooted in this layer and emerging at the *stratum corneum* are hair follicles and sweat glands, crucial to healthy skin.

Key skin components

Sebum (natural skin oil) and moisture are nature's secrets of healthy skin. Sebum forms in tiny glands around every hair on your body. It keeps hairs supple, and it binds the skin's top layer of dead cells, keeping it supple and barricading moisture in, bacteria out. Water is held between all the living cells, nurturing them and giving skin a full, moist look. The skin's own natural humectant, **hyaluronic acid**, attracts water from the air and binds it to the skin.

Sweat, of course, is part of your heat control system; its evaporation cools the body. (Small surface blood capillaries bear away heat, too.) But sweat, along with sebum on the top skin layer, also forms an **acid mantle**. This is a slightly acid film that prevents harmful bacteria from thriving on the skin – your skin is, after all, the first barrier between you and invasive attackers. Chemically speaking, the acid–alkaline balance is called pH. It is rated pH1 for most acid to pH14 to most alkaline, with pH7 at neutral. Skin and hair are naturally pH 5.4–6.2. pH-balanced skin products have a pH of 4: extra protection against bacteria.

Melanin is dark pigment in granules which colour the skin in varying shades of brown from pale to black. The more melanin the darker the skin. Melanin's role is to screen out the sun's ultraviolet (UV) rays which damage the functions of epidermis and dermis. People of Asian, Mediterranean, Latin, African, and Afro-Caribbean ethnic heritage have the natural sun protection developed in their ancestors' original sunny climates. Caucasian skin is less effective at melanin production. (See 'Sunlight', below.)

Key skin enemies

Free radicals are unstable molecules and atoms formed naturally during metabolism. They racket around looking for stability and find it by combining with whatever's around them. This can cause injury, irritation and death to cell parts, cell walls and collagen fibres. In a young, healthy body special natural enzymes and nutrients scavenge and neutralise these wild cards. But sun, air pollution, cigarette smoke, pesticides, poor diet, illness, stress – in short, much of life as we know it – trigger more free radicals than the body's natural defence system can absorb. The result, as far as skin goes, is loss of suppleness, elasticity, resilience, healthiness and ability to self-repair.

Sunlight, not just in the summer by the seaside but all the time, contains UV rays that damage protein fibres, thicken the epidermis and can cause skin cancer. The heat of the sun also robs skin of moisture, promoting dryness and lines. Sunlight offers some advantages – it triggers natural vitamin D production, sometimes helps oily skin and eczema, and it lifts the spirits, possibly due to the light-stimulated hormone, melatonin. (More on sun and tans in Chapter 9.)

Hormones affect sebum production, as any teenager will know. Oestrogen is a natural humectant, influencing the amount of moisture in the skin. As sex hormones decrease with age, skin sebum and moisture decrease.

Environmental heat and dryness Heat, be it from sun or central heating, makes water evaporate from the skin. Cold air, outdoors or from air conditioning, is usually dry and so also dehydrates. Skin's normal sebum and moisture production can't compensate; parched, flaky or cracked skin result.

Poor skincare Products too harsh for your skin type strip sebum and may irritate or scratch skin. Lack of any skin care leaves skin dry and/or ingrained with dirt.

Years gradually slow skin's regeneration ability; new cells take longer to appear, old ones longer to shed. Skin over the muscles controlling smiles and frowns loses protein fibre firmness and elasticity, leaving permanent expression lines and wrinkles. Gravity drags down loose skin.

Health, diet, lifestyle Illness and poor body maintenance patterns affect skin's clarity and functioning. Internal skin nourishment is necessary.

Skincare product lowdown

There's a wealth of products to care for your skin, but 'wealth' need not be interpreted literally: a supermarket or chain pharmacy brand at a low price can work just as effectively as a designer label product at ten times the price. For more background on how the beauty business works, see Chapter 12. Meanwhile, a few basics on skin-product formulation.

Generally, **creams and lotions** consist of oil and water, those natural allies of skin, with an **emulsifier**. The emulsifier (the mineral borax is frequently used) keeps the formula stable and evenly mixed together, otherwise the oil and water would separate, like salad dressing. Beauty manufacturers talk of oil-in-water emulsions, which have more water than oil and tend to be lighter and fluid, or water-in-oil emulsions, which have more oil, so they are heavier, creamier.

The oils (supplementing your own natural sebum, remember) may be less or more refined. Almond and grapeseed oil, for example, are finer than olive oil, and there are varying grades of mineral oil, which comes from petroleum. Waxes (such as beeswax, sheep lanolin, petroleum) are oils in a semi-solid state. They are used in products with stiffer textures, like night creams and lipsticks. Whatever the source and form, oils have what professionals call an **emollient** effect: they lubricate the protein surface of skin to keep it soft and pliable, and to keep moisture in (like wax on shoe leather).

The formulation itself may be more or less refined. Usually the more 'milled' (mixed or ground) a product, the lighter and finer it is. Because it's been through extra processing steps, it's more expensive, and usually more pleasant to use.

Detergents, in **cleansers**, are actually emulsifiers that effectively lift and suspend oil so that water or tissue or cotton wool can easily sweep the mixture away. Dish detergents get food off your crockery this way, but of course they are far harsher than cosmetic detergents.

Gels, made of natural plant or seaweed gums, may substitute for oils in some products. Like oil and emulsifier they keep water and other ingredients in suspension.

Alcohol is used in some products for degreasing and for its astringency, that is, the ability to tighten the skin's surface.

Different formulations suit different skin needs, as well as personal preferences. Other ingredients – **herbal extracts**, **humectants**, **vitamins**, **fruit acids**, **proteins**, etc – are delivered to the skin by the product. **Fragrance** is usually added to make products smell pleasant. If it's a pleasure to use, you'll use it regularly, which means you'll be caring for your skin regularly, which is what's needed to have good skin.

— Your steps to good-looking skin —

The aim of skincare is to keep skin clean and to maintain the crucial blend of oil and water that keeps skin soft, supple and healthy, or to compensate for it, if the balance isn't right. If you are in your twenties with a balanced skin type this can be as simple as one, two: cleanse, moisturise. If your skin isn't quite perfection, four basic steps and some extras will shape it up and keep it looking good.

Tooling-up for skincare

Besides basic warm and cool water and clean towels, you need:

- cotton wool – balls, preshaped pads or tear-off chunks
- tissues
- a stable mirror, ideally in good daylight.

> Always apply skincare products with an upward, outward stroking motion. Don't drag skin down any more than gravity is doing!

Step 1 Cleanse: twice a day

Make-up, dirt from hands, grime from the air, oil from your hair, skin's own sweat, oil and dead cells... if left on your face these block pores, prevent cell shedding, can build up and irritate skin and attract further dirt and bacteria. Without regular, twice-daily cleansing skin becomes unhealthy. Furthermore, dirt can prevent other skincare products from working efficiently. Generally, morning cleansing can be quicker and lighter than the evening removal of a day's dirt and make-up. You can use the same products morning and evening, or choose two different routines.

Cleansing creams, milks

Oil based, with more or less water content depending on the product you choose, these dissolve the oils from make-up and from your own skin build-up. A cleanser should glide quickly and easily over the skin, allowing you to massage skin and wipe away cleanser with tissues or cotton wool. Some cleansers are designed to be splashed away, a nice compromise for water lovers. It's more effective to cleanse twice with smaller amounts than once with a big glob.

Ideal for: dry, balanced, combination, sensitive or mature skin. The drier or more mature the skin type, the richer (creamier) the cleanser should be.

Cleansing lotions, bars

Soapless pH-balanced detergents that lather with water are not ideal for make-up removal as they contain no oil, but they do degrease skin. Great for soap-and-water lovers, these special 'soaps' are far better for your face than normal bath soap which is a detergent so strong that it strips skin oils harshly, leaving skin feeling tight and dry. What's more, in oily skin, too harsh cleansing can stimulate even more oil production. Splashing your face with lots of water to rinse helps the cleansing operation, but not if your water is hard; it leaves a film on skin like it does on your basin.

Ideal for: oily, balanced, combination or troubled skin.

Eye make-up remover

This fine oil or very mild detergent lotion floats away eye make-up, especially stubborn mascara. For waterproof mascara, oil-based remover is required. Apply gently with finger tips or cotton wool, wipe away with tissue or cotton wool. Wait a few moments before wiping away to let the product act. Do not pull or rub hard at the eye area; skin here is very thin and fragile.

Ideal for: eye make-up wearers. Don't go around with smudges under your eyes!

Step 2 Tone: after cleansing

Called tonics, bracers, fresheners, lotions, under a variety of names skin toners contain from 50 per cent to 10 per cent alcohol. Basically water and alcohol, perhaps with plant extracts, fruit acids or other ingredients, a toner completes the cleansing process, especially when you use oil-based cleansers. It helps to restore the skin's bacteria-fighting pH balance and it astringes (closes the pores) after any kind of cleansing, massage or heat treatment. Apply with cotton wool; reapply until the cotton comes away clean. The rubbing action mildly exfoliates skin, a bonus benefit.

Ideal for: all skin types, especially oily and those who use creamy, milky cleansers. The drier your skin, the lower the alcohol content should be.

Step 3 Exfoliate: once or twice a week

Considered part of the cleansing process, exfoliation is the removal of dead, surface skin cells. Skin sheds cells naturally as new cells push up, but the rate is accelerated in dark Asian and black skin types, and slows with the years in other skin types. Exfoliants help slough off the dead cells to prevent dullness and pore blockage, brightening the complexion and giving it a healthy freshness.

Don't be overenthusiastic in exfoliating or you may irritate or overstimulate skin. Black skin is prone to scarring, so use refined products and go gently. Follow exfoliation with toning and/or other occasional deep beauty treatments. You have a choice of exfoliating methods, as follows.

Scrubs, pads

A scrub is essentially a cleanser with little grains of walnut shell, oatmeal, silica or other tiny bits in it. Mildly abrasive to rub away dead cells, it should be massaged over skin after cleansing and usually rinsed away with water. Special buffing pads perform the same function.

Ideal for: balanced, oily, combination (especially in the T-zone) skin.

Peeling masks

These may be gels, or creams with clay; some stiffen on the skin. Gentler than scrubs, they absorb grime and oil and may contain mild organic peeling agents. The action of peeling away the mask takes away the dead cells.

Ideal for: all skin types, especially dry, black, mature and sensitive.

Step 4 Moisturise: twice a day

The key to soft, smooth skin is water; natural skin oils help to keep water inside the skin, but even putting extra water on your face can't make water stay in the skin. Dryness and heat (see 'Key skin enemies', page 42) pull water out. So, as well as oil and water, moisturising products contain a humectant – a water attractor that helps to keep moisture in skin's upper layers. The oils lubricate the skin surface, and also help prevent moisture escaping from deeper skin layers.

Moisturiser for morning: lotions, milks, creams

Usually fluid oil-in-water emulsions, these smooth on and soak into skin quickly. Creams are richer and leave a slight surface film for better defence. Look for moisturisers with sunscreens to protect against UVA and UVB rays. Moisturiser provides an even base for foundation make-up, allowing it to spread and blend well and stopping pores from filling with make-up. Tinted moisturisers give both protection and light colour.

Ideal for: all skin types. Choose a moisturiser that you enjoy using and use it every day after morning cleansing. Adapt to richer products as you grow older, if you're exposed to hot or cold dry air. If you're under age 22 or have oily skin you may not need a moisturiser, but you should still use sunscreen.

Night moisturiser: creams

Because skin renews itself most actively as you sleep, it's best to use a richer moisturiser at bedtime. Night creams are usually water-in-oil emulsions, so they are highly emollient, softening skin and keeping it elastic. They contain humectants and often other ingredients to soothe and nourish skin.

Ideal for: all but the oiliest skin types. If you have younger and oily skin, even balanced skin, you may prefer to use your day moisturiser by night. As you get older or if you have dry or mature skin, use richer creams to make up for sebum reduction.

Step 5 Extras: special treatments, if needed

Facial masks: weekly or as needed

A face mask can deep-cleanse skin and stimulate microcirculation, and it can help many specific problems, depending on the mask and its active ingredients. Generally you apply the mask, avoiding eye area, wait 10 to 20 minutes, then remove. Use the waiting time to lie back and rest, or to attend to your hairy legs or pedicure. There are three basic mask formulations; follow manufacturers' guidelines as to which mask to use for what purpose.

Non-setting masks – creamy or gel, often to refresh and deep-moisturise skin; usually wipe away.

Setting masks – usually made with clay or calamine which draws impurities from skin, they dry and harden; removal usually with water.

Peel-off masks – wax, gum, latex or plastic bases have various cleansing effects; gels cool. They stiffen; pull or roll the mask off.

Ideal for: all skin types. Don't answer the door while using one! You can use problem-specific masks in problem areas only, say deep cleansing for oily T-zone, or deep moisturising for flaky cheeks. Blemishes may emerge during two days following a cleansing mask – this is a good sign: it's toxins coming out. Skin will calm by day three and look great.

Anti-wrinkle creams: as needed

Extra rich in oils, these products with names that suggest they combat wrinkles are actually moisturisers. They may have finer oils and waxes than normal moisturisers; they contain humectants, water, and probably herbs, fruit acids or similar active ingredients to stimulate circulation and sloughing of dead cells. Some contain collagen or elastin, which are protein fibres like those in the dermis; these are good humectants, but they probably don't do anything directly for your own skin proteins. Every few years there's a new 'wonder' ingredient or formulation (once antioxidants, then liposomes were the hot new thing, AHAs are the discovery of the 90s – see 'Miracle claims', Chapter 12). Any effect, even when ingredient action is genuine, is subtle. Major wrinkles – crow's feet, smile lines, forehead expression lines – may be subtly plumped, but they can't be erased. Crepey, parched skin can, however, improve with good moisturising.

Ideal for: those who can afford them. Otherwise, just step up your exfoliation routine and try a richer-than-normal moisturiser. If wrinkly skin really bothers you, see 'Major changes', Chapter 11.

Eyecare: nightly as needed

These very lightweight creams or gels are simply ultra-refined moisturisers. Skin around the eyes is very thin, with scant fatty layers and sebaceous glands, so this area gets dehydrated easily and develops lines and wrinkles early. Beneath the eyes, skin thins with age, fatigue, illness or simply genetic heritage: the microcirculation blood supply shows through as reddish-blue circles. Puffy eyes mean the skin is congested and retaining fluid – tiredness, allergies, toxins, sinus problems or greasy creams can be causes.

Eye creams help to plump out dryness and tiny wrinkles without blocking pores or dragging on skin. Eye gels or lotions cool and reduce puffiness. Both kinds of formulation may contain mild herbs which aid circulation and healing. A light moisturiser will probably do the same job. Whichever you use, apply with a finger, gently dotting and patting into skin; don't rub.

Ideal for: those who can afford them. Worth a try by late-night socialisers, exam crammers, mothers of non-sleeping infants, those in their thirties and beyond.

Neck creams: nightly as needed, but ...

These are moisturisers, fine and rich in texture because neck skin is thin and unsupported, rather like eye-area skin. People often forget their necks when cleansing and moisturising, yet your neck shows almost as much as your face. And it is certainly exposed to ageing sunrays. Instead of using specific neck cream you can use your daytime, sun-screened moisturiser, your own basic night cream or an anti-wrinkle cream.

Ideal for: those who can afford them. However, if buying a neck cream makes you remember to care for your neck, then it's worth it to you.

Skincare specifics

As well as having basically dry, oily, combination or balanced skin, you may have occasional or additional special skin problems. Here's what to do ...

Black/dark Asian skin

Though faithful cleansing and exfoliating is vital because this skin type sheds cells rapidly, do not make the mistake of using harsh products. Dark skin readily scars, so treat it gently. Resist the temptation to lighten dark patches or your entire complexion – skin bleaches can irritate and leave permanent blotches.

Try: cleansing milk rather than lathering cleanser; non-alcoholic or mild toner; light, non-greasy moisturising lotion. Exfoliate gently twice weekly, mask twice weekly to help prevent dead skin-cell build-up. Rich night creams aren't necessary; use your day moisturiser at night.

Sensitive skin

If you get rashes, redness, dryness, stinging, etc, discontinue use of your main current product and try a substitute. Keep going until you eliminate the culprit. Irritability or allergic reactions are more common in dry skin, but anyone might get them. Be sure your diet is balanced; keep up your water intake.

What to do: Handle skin carefully. Seek products labelled for sensitive skin. These are usually formulated without fragrance and other ingredients known to irritate particularly sensitive skin. Using deep-moisturising masks may help; don't use hard-setting clay masks.

Dehydrated skin

Anyone's skin, even the oiliest, can get dry and flaky now and then. It could be due to climate changes in seasons, and visiting places hotter, drier or colder than you are used to. It could also be due to incorrect skincare: cleanser or toner too harsh, exfoliant or mask too stimulating, moisturiser not rich enough.

What to do: Check your products. A deep-moisturising mask is very helpful.

Troubled skin

Pimples, blackheads, whiteheads, blocked pores, possible inflammation, swelling and lumpy texture: all these are usually the woes of excessively oily skin, although anyone can have a spot now and then (usually due to sex hormone swings). Then there's acne and its older lookalike, rosacea.

For all troubled skin: Look for anti-bacterial products with ingredients that help prevent infection spreading. Avoid touching your face; keep hair away from your face.

How to handle a pimple: Don't! Certainly do not squeeze a headless pimple. It's best just to dab on an anti-bacterial liquid and leave it alone to heal. A pustule (as professionals call it) is a raised, inflamed spot on the skin which contains pus. If pus is visible, then you may – carefully – hurry a pimple's resolution. Cleanse your face, cleanse the area with an alcoholic toner. With clean hands and a clean tissue gently squeeze out the pimple head. Dab area gently with anti-bacterial toner on cotton wool. Never squeeze at a headless pimple; you risk spreading infection deep and wide.

How to handle a blackhead: A comedone, as it is called by professionals, is sebum trapped in a hair follicle by a plug made of dead skin cells and exposed, hardened sebum. Cleanse, then steam your face (see 'Steam treatment' later in this chapter), use clean fingers and a tissue to squeeze out the plug. A blackhead-extracting tool might help. It's best to attack blackheads over several sessions, to avoid damaging skin. Follow each session with toner to tighten the pores. Instead or as well, try a specially-for-blackheads mask-type product.

How to handle a whitehead: Milia (the professional name) are small pearl-like bumps made when a thin layer of skin grows over the end of a hair follicle or sweat gland. They often occur in low oil-producing areas of the face. After cleanser and alcohol-based toner, use a sterile needle gently to prick the skin over the whitehead, then squeeze out the hardened deposit. Clean again with alcoholic or anti-bacterial tonic.

How to handle acne: Acne is due to a chain of events. Hormone imbalance makes sebaceous glands overactive; bacteria in hair follicles attack the sebum; this leads to irritation of the follicle, then blockage and eventual rupture of the sebum gland within the dermis (see skin diagram). Inflammation and infection of the sebum gland follow, and the resulting angry bumpiness of acne. Experts now say that chocolate and fatty food do not provoke acne. Scrupulous cleansing and anti-bacterial products are essential; sunshine seems to help, too. Don't use very drying products as irritated skin can block follicles, making the problem worse. Steam and squeeze headed pimples, as above, **only** if spots are not red and painful. See a doctor for antibiotics if the problem is severe. Unfortunately acne can only be controlled, not cured; it can last eight years or longer, reaching a peak at about age 17, improving and ceasing in the mid-twenties. If scarring is worrisome, medical cosmetic treatment may help – see Chapter 11.

How to handle rosacea: This bright reddening of nose and cheeks can appear from thirty-something up to the menopause. It usually begins with temporary flushing in response to alcohol, spicy food, hot drinks or hot environments. The flushing then becomes permanent as capillaries remain dilated. This extra blood flow in turn stimulates sebum production which leads to bumps, pimples and coarse pores, as for acne. Treat as for acne, including antibiotics if necessary. Rosacea is a chronic disorder that lasts for five to ten years, then disappears.

Ageing and mature skin

Ageing skin – and this generally occurs from mid-thirties on – benefits from extra care, more so as you enter the late forties and fifties, around and after the menopause. Rich and stimulating treatments improve skin texture and fine dryness wrinkles, although they cannot alter crow's feet, deep expression lines, sagging jowls and eye bags. If you're distressed by dramatic signs of ageing, maybe your answer is professional intervention (see below, and Chapter 11). Serum-based products can give an instant lift; they dry to a taut film (rather like egg white) but they leave you with a stiff, artificial face, and last only briefly.

Mature skin, of the seventies and eighties, is thin, dry and translucent, has lost its firmness, is 'quilted' with lines. Cleansing, stimulation and rich moisturising will keep skin refined and fresh-looking.

What to do: Use richer creams; step up exfoliation and stimulating masks to promote skin regeneration, warm oil masks to deep moisturise. Don't regret your wrinkles; every one of them has a history of laughter, tears, talk, smiles, life.

Other troubles

Unwanted facial hair

Never shave – hair grows back with blunt ends that look coarse and stubbly. Bleaching is the easiest way to fade out downy hair; results last a month and you can do it at home. Use tweezers to pluck out coarse individual hairs. If growth is heavy, chemical depilatories dissolve hair (dangerous to do on the face at home), waxing pulls it out by the roots. These two methods are best done by a salon. A professional can remove hair with electrolysis – this kills the hair root with an elecric current via a fine needle; it usually takes a course of sessions, and can be expensive and painful, but it's permanent.

Broken capillaries

These occur when walls of the tiny blood vessels weaken due to fine skin or harsh treatment; blood leaks into surrounding tissue or capillaries radiate out in a spider-leg pattern. Diathermy can make this problem disappear; it's electricity delivered through a fine needle which cauterises the vessels and harmlessly blocks off the blood flow. Find an electrologist at a good salon, via a dermatologist, or see Chapter 11.

Birthmarks, moles, skin tags, scars

These can sometimes be removed very easily (see Chapter 11); if not, good camouflage make-up can help (see Chapter 8).

Home-based skincare recipes

Steam treatment Heat is the essence of many professional, deep cleansing and nourishing treatments which you can replicate at home. Cleanse your face. Use a bowl or the bathroom basin; pour boiling water over five to ten camomile teabags (it's a naturally healing herb). Drape a towel over your head and lean over the steam for ten minutes or so. Blot your face dry. Extract any blackheads or ready pimples. Finish with toner and then moisturiser.

Cleanser Use baby oil or lotion to lift off make-up, grime and oils.

Toner Buy plain rosewater and plain witch hazel from a pharmacy. Mix one quarter witch hazel to three-quarters rosewater in a clean bottle. For oilier skin, increase the proportion of witch hazel, for drier skin, decrease.

Moisturiser Petroleum jelly functions just like an expensive cream. It seals moisture in and lubricates the surface. Of course it does not contain sunscreen, humectants, healing or stimulating botanicals or fragrance, and it does not quickly 'soak in' to the skin. However, if you really want to save money and avoid hype, it does the job that needs to be done.

Deep moisture treatment Snip a capsule of evening primrose oil and smooth over skin.

Exfoliation Take a handful of fine oatmeal, ground almonds and/or bran, stir into two to three tablespoons of plain yogurt. Use immediately on clean skin; rinse and tone afterwards. Also, when you bathe, give your face a gentle go with your washing flannel or towel to scuff away dead skin cells.

Eye pack Fresh cucumber slices, or cooled, used teabags – place on eyelids and lie back and listen to peaceful music. Reduces puffiness and soreness.

Facial masks Mayonnaise provides a deep moisturising treatment, or try avocado mashed with a little olive oil and honey. For a cleansing mask, mix plain yogurt and fine oatmeal into a paste, add a little lemon juice and some grated carrot or puréed parsley.

Making faces

Simple exercises will aid your complexion by stimulating the facial microcirculation that feeds and cleans the deep skin layers where new skin cells are formed.

The lion

Scrunch up every muscle in your face as tightly as you can – eyes squeezed, eyebrows frowned, mouth pursed, jaw clenched. Hold, then open everything as wide as you can, include your tongue, sticking it out and down as far as you can. Repeat two or three times. It looks demented, so do it privately.

Shoulder stand

(Before doing this check with your doctor if you have a heart or blood condition.)

Lie flat on the floor on your back, arms at your sides, palms down. Lift your legs slowly straight up, so you form an L-shape. Now press your palms into the floor and roll your waist and hips from the floor, so your feet begin to reach over your head. Prop your hands against your back for support and slowly straighten your legs so they point towards the ceiling (or as nearly straight as you can get). Hold this position for 30 seconds. Throughout this you must continue to breathe slowly and steadily.

To descend, lower your knees slowly towards your head. Put your arms and hands back on the floor and roll your back and waist slowly down to the floor; keep your head on the floor. Now straighten your knees so you are L-shaped again, then slowly lower your straight legs to the floor. Let your body go limp.

Finger pressure face massage

Give yourself a fingertip facial based on the oriental shiatsu technique illustrated and described in Chapter 10. It promotes lymph and blood circulation, and releases the muscle tension that can create a strained, lined look.

Complete Yoga Breath

The extra oxygen exchange of conscious deep breathing brings vitality to the skin. See 'Get a lungful' instructions in Chapter 3.

What a professional can do for you

Is beauty salon treatment worth the time and expense? Sensible French women visit their skin clinics as often or more than they do their hairdressers – and French skin and style show it. Approach salon care with the notion of a series of treatments. A one-off will be pleasurable, but a series – say a visit every two to four weeks for a season – will build up the benefits so improvement really shows.

You can do many treatments for yourself at home, but a salon offers:

- **Knowledge:** different areas of the face and special problems get attention from an expert qualified in physiology and product use. She can alert you to a need for medical attention if she spots a problem.
- **Thoroughness:** every pore is examined; a therapist may use a dozen products on you; a full facial lasts over an hour.
- **Professional massage:** therapists' massage techniques stimulate circulation, relax muscles. Neck and upper shoulder areas are included in facials. Great for stress as well as skin, hands-on care is not to be belittled if your lifestyle crowds out your own needs for nurturing.
- **High technology:** brushes, steamers, extractors, electrical equipment. Vacuum suction, for instance, aids lymphatic drainage and microcirculation. In facial galvanic electrical treatment a current propels special products into the skin. In facial faradic electrical treatment a current makes muscles contract and relax, to firm sagging skin contours – some muscles you just can't exercise yourself. The lifting and tightening can have a visible (temporary) effect.
- **Other services:** electrologist, waxing, manicure, pedicure, make-up.

LIVING FOR SKIN

- Drink lots of water.
- Eat healthily. Lots more fresh vegetables, fruit, fibre than processed, sugary and fatty foods.
- The skin vitamins and minerals are: A, B, C, E, calcium, copper, iron, zinc.
- No smoking; it leathers skin.
- Cut down on alcohol: flushes complexion, enlarges pores.
- Get your beauty sleep; it's when skin regenerates.
- Exercise the whole body, especially aerobically.

5

THE SHINING: HAIR

Whatever the cut, style and colour, great-looking hair is shining clean and in good condition. Here's the know-how you need to manage and care for your hair.

Ten-step self-assessment: what's your hair profile?

As you read through the ten steps below, tick the hair type which applies to you.

Step 1 Your natural base colour

- fair – light blonde to dark blonde
- brown – light brown to dark brown
- dark – very dark brown to black
- red – pale strawberry to ginger to auburn
- grey – white to steel to salt-and-pepper

Step 2 Your natural tone

Most colours have subtle undertones or tinges. Examine a strand of your hair in good daylight; is it:

- ashen, cool
- golden, yellow
- warm, ruddy?

Step 3   Your natural abundance

How many hairs per square centimetre do you have? Don't count them, but is your hair:

- thin in coverage
- medium thickness
- thick, abundant?

Step 4   Your natural texture

Each individual hair is:

- fine
- medium
- coarse?

Step 5   Your hair's 'alpha keratin' state

This describes its natural behaviour. Is it:

- straight – Oriental, Asian, others
- wavy – gentle curves to near-curls
- curly – mild corkscrews to tight curls
- kinky – Afro-Caribbean, each strand is bumpy?

Step 6   Your hair's natural sebaceousness

Sebum production from the scalp coats hair. Is yours:

- dry – needs washing no more than once or twice a week
- balanced – needs washing two or three times a week
- oily – needs washing daily or every other day?

Step 7   Your scalp

Is it naturally:

- dry – perhaps occasional flakiness
- balanced – no problems
- oily – usually goes with oily complexion
- oily or dry with dandruff?

Step 8 Your hair's condition

Is your hair generally:

- shining, smooth
- dry, dull, porous – sun or chemical damage
- troubled with split ends, does it tangle easily – physical or chemical damage?

Steps 9 and 10

Now for two close-up professional tests of hair condition, best done on clean, towel-dried hair. Don't worry, whatever your hair profile, help is at hand.

Elasticity
With thumb and forefinger pinch a small lock of hair near the ends and gently pull, then let go. Healthy hair should stretch about half its length when wet (one-third when dry), then return to its original length. This quality of elasticity gives hair its spring and bounciness. Hair that stretches more than this is over-elastic. Without help it can become limp, lifeless and in danger of breaking off.

Porosity
Hold one or several hairs at the far end, slide your other fingers along the strand towards the roots. This goes against the grain of the cuticle scales: the rougher it feels, the more damaged hair is. Porous hair quickly or unevenly absorbs water or chemicals into the hair shaft; without special care you risk frizziness, breakage or patchy colour.

Hair know-how: what is hair?

To understand the structure and life of your hair is to know how to manage it. Strange to think, all the hair that you see is dead – it is made of the protein **keratin**, which is produced in hair **follicles** in the dermis layer of your scalp. If you look at the skin diagram in Chapter 4 you'll see that each hair has its own sebaceous gland which produces natural oils (sebum) to lubricate the hair and skin to keep them supple, smooth and protected. Too much **sebum** results in oiliness, too little means dry skin and hair. The purpose of hair, biologically speaking, is to protect the scalp from burning and to retain body heat; it's also a social and sexual signal, which is why we care about it so much.

Your head has 100,000 to 150,000 hairs on it. Redheads generally have the the fewest hairs, but each strand is thicker; blondes usually have the most hairs, but the strands are finer: you win some, you lose some in this hair game. And we all do lose some, an average of 100 hairs a day. This is because each hair has a **life growth cycle**. For about three to five years new cells are constantly produced at the hair root at the bottom of the follicle. Here in the dermis tiny blood capillaries deliver oxygen and nutrients and take away waste to nourish this growth. At the rate of about 1.25 cm ($^1/_2$ inch) per month the new cells are pushed upwards and hardened to become the hair we see. But at some stage, each follicle rests; it shrinks and stops cell production for three or four months. When growth begins again the new hair pushes out the old hair forcing it to shed. Fortunately follicles aren't synchronised, so you don't shed all your hair at the same time and go bald.

RAPUNZEL, RAPUNZEL

My friend can sit on her hair, but mine never grows below my shoulders ...

This means that your friend has hair with a long life cycle – it grows for something like 7 years at 1.25 cm ($^1/_2$ inch) per month. So each hair can grow to 105 cm (42 inches) before it drops out at the end of its seven-year life.

Yours might grow for only 1 year at 1.25 cm ($^1/_2$ inch) per month before it stops. So each hair only grows to 15 cm (6 inches) before it sheds after its one-year life. Take heart, hair with a short life cycle is likely to have fewer split ends.

More hair growth facts

- Hair can grow at different rates in different places on the head.
- Hair grows faster when heat from summer sun or exercise improves microcirculation to the hair follicles.
- The hormones oestrogen and progesterone affect hair quality – sometimes for better, sometimes not.

Hair structure

Now as to the structure of the hair itself: like a pencil, it has three layers.

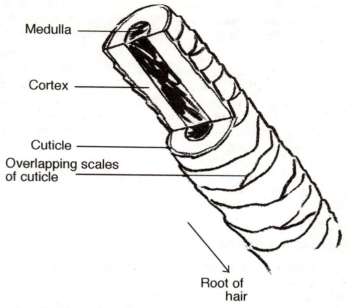

Figure 5 Hair health: a cross-section

The *centre layer* (imagine the pencil's lead) is called the **medulla** and has little function.

The *thick surrounding layer* (imagine the pencil's wood), called the **cortex**, consists of many fibres of the protein keratin, all twisted together. The cortex is the hair's source of colour and curl.

Colour comes from the pigments **melanin** (brown/black) and **pheomelanin** (yellow/red) scattered in various amounts in the cortex. Medium-brown hair has lots of brown and a little black, red and yellow pigment, while coppery red hair has lots of red, some yellow and a little brown and black pigment, and so forth. White or grey hair has no pigments.

Curl comes from the keratin protein bonds in the cortex. Your hair when natural, dry and untreated (virgin) is in its **alpha keratin state**. When it is reshaped by wetting, stretching and heat (for example, blow-drying, setting on rollers) or perms it is in a **beta keratin state**. Some of the protein bonds are temporary – water weakens them, drying reforms them, so your blow-dry or set lasts until moisture breaks the bonds again. Hair also has permanent protein bonds which can be broken only by a strong chemical, which is how perms work to hold curl.

The *outer layer* of a hair's structure is the thin, flat **cuticle** (imagine the paint on a pencil). It's made up of overlapping **scales** of keratin, rather like roof tiles, all lying away from the scalp. Healthy, tight-closed, flat scales make hair shiny and smooth, protecting the cortex. Perms and bleaches have to open up the scales to do their work in the cortex, so, unless properly conditioned, cuticle scales remain raised and hair looks and feels rough and dull. Exposure to sun, heat, chlorine, sea water, harsh shampooing, back-brushing and tight elastics can also damage the cuticle. Damaged scales mean hair is porous and vulnerable because moisture and chemicals (colour, perms) can easily get to the cortex.

Hair management facts

'Bad hair days' happen because hair is **hygroscopic** – it absorbs water from the atmosphere. Does your hairstyle go flat and limp in a fog, or wild and frizzy on rainy days? It's because the cuticle scales open and the bonds of your well-behaved, blow-dried beta keratin hairstyle return to their natural alpha keratin state. Styling products keep those scales closed to keep moisture out. It's a case of 'Water, stay away from my beta keratin bonds!'

Playing pHair   The natural, protective acid–alkaline balance of hair and scalp is pH 4.5 to 5.5. This is slightly acid (water, at pH 7, is exactly neutral). **Alkalis** open cuticle scales, which can be useful: tints and bleaches are pH 8.6 to 9.2, perms are pH 9.5, relaxers used on Afro-Caribbean hair are pH 10 to 14. On the other hand, **acid-balanced** products keep cuticle scales closed, hair smooth and shining: conditioners are pH 4 to 6.

Electric hair   Just like fibres in a carpet or a sweater, your individual hairs have an electrical charge, positive or negative. If it's too much one way or the other, which may happen with the friction of brushing or drying, positive repels positive or negative repels negative, and the result is fly-away hair. Conditioners and mousse products, like laundry conditioners for sweaters, restore electrical balance, keeping hair calm and soft.

Haircare product lowdown

A **shampoo** is a specially formulated **mild detergent** which lifts and envelops particles of dirt and grease with minimal ruffling of cuticle scales. The grubby bits are floated away by floods of rinse water. Dishwashing detergent works on the same principle, but it's made to work on food and cooking grease; soap is even harsher and leaves a residue. Generally, more expensive shampoos contain finer, gentler or richer, more costly ingredients, and bottom-of-the-price-range shampoos are pretty basic – but they work in the same way. Somehow the fragrance and the amount of lather make you feel that a particular shampoo is better than others, but these two factors are strictly 'cosmetic', a matter of personal preference – and why not? Hair-washing is a sensual experience.

Hair shampoos usually also contain some oils and other ingredients for special needs. Your hair may like or not like one shampoo or another – you'll quickly tell by its behaviour and feel. Experiment with shampoo by using travel sizes, free samples and sachets. Shampoo formulae vary; for special hair problems, see 'Haircare specifics' later in this chapter.

Regular shampoos: for balanced, dry or oily hair; frequent-use shampoos clean more mildly.

Treatment shampoos: for instance, medicated, for dandruff, or with proteins for porous, damaged hair.

Specialist shampoos: for example, clarifying deep-cleanser to remove built-up sticky layers on overconditioned or heavily styled hair.

Two-in-one shampoos/conditioners: convenient for taking to gym, pool, tennis, seaside, etc. On a regular basis this kind of conditioning may cling too heavily or not do enough for your hair.

Conditioners contain **oils** to lubricate keratin and allow cuticle scales to stay supple and closed, guarding against moisture imbalance, roughness and tangling. The light coating of oil also banishes static electricity. Look for acid-balanced conditioners to keep cuticles closed. Vitamins, proteins and other ingredients may be able to help damaged hair if they can penetrate through the porous cuticle to the cortex (see specific hair needs, below). There are different types of conditioners; manufacturers' guidance, trial use and your hairdresser's advice will help you decide which to use.

Instant rinse-away conditioners: generally these are creamy lotions that lightly coat and smooth the cuticle; you apply to towel-blotted hair every time you shampoo, leave five minutes and rinse well.

Leave-in conditioners: sprays, creams, mousse, etc. you apply after your regular shampoo, comb through and don't rinse away. Good on greasy, fine, tangled or kinky hair.

Deep conditioners: dry hair benefits from an occasional dose of oil (usually almond, coconut, etc). or rich cream conditioner. These treatment packs are usually helped by heat – follow package instructions.

Specialist deep reconditioners: may be single-dose sachets, thick cream in jars, thin serum, mousse ... these can rescue poor, weak, overexposed or overprocessed hair. Used over four to six weeks, they are generally applied once a week after shampoo, then rinsed out. Restructurants, with protein, are usually not rinsed out.

Dry-use conditioners: not for wet hair, you apply a tiny amount of this rich cream with your palms, or spray on a whisper of fine oil after drying and styling or any time. These condition, shine and calm flyaway or frizzy hair.

— Your steps to good-looking hair —

The aim of haircare is to keep the hair and scalp clean, and hair itself shining and manageable. One essential ingredient is the haircut – we look at hairstyles in Chapter 7 – but whatever the look, regular haircuts (every four to eight weeks) trim away damaged ends to keep hair healthy. Meanwhile, there's plenty to do at home ...

Tooling-up for haircare

As well as hot and cold running water and, ideally, a good showerhead (alternatively a plastic jug), and absorbent towels, you need:

- hair brush – firm, plentiful, flexible bristles to allow thorough grooming of scalp and hair
- wide-toothed comb – or 'rake' comb, for detangling wet hair
- normal comb – for sectioning and styling hair.

Step 1 Shampoo for clean hair

Clean hair smells good and it feels good. Even the act of shampooing itself is a kind of mini-renewal. Washing removes the build-up of airborne dirt, oil (sebum) from hair follicles, dead skin cells from the scalp, and coatings of hair spray, mousse, gel or other styling products.

How often to shampoo? As often as it looks or feels in need; this might be once a week or once a day. You should be a more frequent shampooer if you have oily scalp and hair, or if you use lots of hairstyling products. Basically, wash before hair gets lank, limp, dull, heavy, and/or scalp gets itchy, flakey. There's no excuse for poor hair hygiene.

Shampooing guidance

For choice of shampoo, see 'Haircare product lowdown', earlier in this chapter. Pour some shampoo into the palm of your hand and apply to wet hair and scalp in several places, then massage it over your head with the flat of your fingertips. Most people (and shampoo manufacturers) prefer two sudsings, although it's not strictly necessary, and not a good idea if your hair is very oily, very dry or very frequently washed. Make your final rinse really thorough so no residue remains to dull the hair.

Pre-shampoo tip: See 'A brush with destiny', p. 71.

End-shampoo tip: The final rinse should be with the shower spray or jugs of cool, fresh water to help cuticles close up.

Budget shampoo tip: You can dilute shampoo with water in your palm or in the bottle as it empties. Most formulations are concentrated and will work just as well 'thinned out'. Want to use a deluxe shampoo? Save by washing hair first with a basic brand, use the more refined one for your second lathering.

Emergency shampoo tip: Oily hair, fringe and no time? Try shampooing and styling the fringe alone for a short-cut to freshness.

Ill, stranded, caught off guard or out of time? Try a dry shampoo. Either sprinkle talc or baby powder on hair and brush through (this absorbs oils). Or dampen cotton wool with an alcohol product (cologne, body fragrance, complexion toner) and dab at roots and along the length of hair (this dissolves oils).

Step 2 Detangle and condition for smooth hair

After shampooing and rinsing, blot your hair with a towel; don't rub and scrub at it – it is stretched out, elastic and vulnerable when wet. If your hair is perfectly healthy, shiny and manageable (which probably means you are under 12 years old), you may not wish to condition it, so the next step is to comb it through gently with a wide-toothed comb to smooth out tangles. It's important to hold a lock of hair a short distance from the hair ends and comb out the ends first, so you don't pull at the hair roots and risk breaking or tearing out hair.

If your hair is not in ideal shape, you can condition it into health and good behaviour. The right conditioning can restore bounce, shine, body and manageability to damaged or misbehaving hair. In short, it can work a miracle – except it doesn't last. Remember, the hair you see is dead and can't be repaired permanently, so you have to condition regularly to keep up the perfect look. Without conditioning, hair damage gets worse. For choice of conditioners and how they're used, see 'Haircare product lowdown' earlier in this chapter. Always be sure to rinse rinse-out conditioners thoroughly.

Drippy conditioning tip: Too-wet hair dilutes conditioner, makes it less effective; be sure to towel-dry hair.

Focus conditioning tip: Avoid putting conditioner on scalp, concentrate on the rest of the hair length. Apply generously to the most exposed and vulnerable areas – hair ends and front hairline.

Hectic conditioning tip: In a hurry in the shower? Instead of the usual 'blot dry, apply conditioner and leave it on for five to ten minutes' routine, you can shampoo, squeeze out excess water, be generous with conditioner and wash the rest of you during the 'wait' period, rinsing out conditioner just before you leave the shower.

Mama bear conditioning tip: Hair gone too soft and unmanageable? Could be your conditioner's too nourishing; change brands to find one that's just right.

Holiday conditioning tip: That paradise island may be hell on hair. If the sun and the frequent pool and sea plunges frazzle your hair, don't rinse out conditioner applied after every shampoo. The next swim will rinse it away.

Haircare specifics

Split ends, dull, rough?

It's too bad that the things we do to give ourselves a hairstyle we like, such as perm, tint or bleach, chemically harm hair. And a healthy, active lifestyle – wind, sun, swimming – also wreaks havoc. Your hair can become so dry, the cuticle so open and porous, that the hair ends split like old, frayed rope. The best cure is a haircut, trimming to a length where hair is healthier. Then start a programme of specialist deep reconditioners or, for slightly less drastic damage, deep oil conditioners. If hair is very damaged or breaking off, consult a hairdresser.

Lank, heavy, dull, sticky?

Maybe your hair is oily and simply needs more frequent washing, a hormonal fact of life for many teenagers and some mums to be. Or it could be that you are not adequately rinsing out your conditioner. Sticky build-up can also be caused by an over-rich conditioner or an excess of styling products. Vary products and routines; you also may need a specialist clarifying shampoo to remove the build-up.

Combination situation: dry hair, oily scalp?

This comes about with oily hair that has been damaged and has dry ends, or sometimes with dandruff that soaks up the natural oils and prevents them from lubricating the length of the hair in the normal way. Treat the dandruff, if any (see below). Use mild shampoo (for normal hair or babies); condition the ends only – keep conditioner away from the scalp.

Dandruff

Snowy shoulders, a flakey hair parting – who needs it! Oily or dry, most dandruff is caused by a fungal yeast that makes scalp skin cells accelerate their replacement cycle, clump together and form flakes. Another version is seborrheoic dermatitis, most common in men, when a red, scaly, itchy rash develops on nose, eyebrows and scalp. Brush hair regularly to loosen flakes. Twice a week for two to four weeks, use special dandruff shampoo medicated to combat the cause; active ingredients that help include selinium sulphide, zinc pyrithione and ketoconazole. After lathering, let the shampoo rest on the scalp for a few minutes before rinsing. Once dandruff is cleared, go back to your usual shampoo, and use the dandruff shampoo once every two weeks in a maintenance programme. Consult your pharmacist or doctor if dandruff persists.

Afro-Caribbean hair

African and Afro-Caribbean hair is much drier and more fragile than other hair types. It tends to tangle easily because of its curl and crinkliness; ends may even be damaged or broken by simply combing and brushing through tangles. Use shampoos which have mild detergents and extra moisturising and detangling ingredients. Follow with an oil-based conditioner for hair *and* scalp. Treated or damaged hair needs penetrating conditioners with special protein moisture agents.

White hair

Whether it's a few silver threads or a whole pure white headful, the texture of white hair is usually coarse and porous, which means it needs a rich and cuticle-binding conditioner. If your white hair is just growing in, tame it by trying out new conditioners to keep hair shiny.

Thinning hair or bald patches

Some kind of hair loss affects up to half of all women as well as men at some point in their lives, and the psychological and social impact can be devastating. The loss happens because of an interruption in the hair-growth life cycle – new growth is scarce or ceases altogether. This, of course, is the reason for hair loss in chemotherapy; when the body recovers from the massive life-saving doses of drugs the hair cycle recovers, too, and growth begins again.

Hair loss occurs in everyday life, often because hormones interrupt the hair-growth life cycle. Pregnancy, childbirth, starting or stopping the contraceptive pill may bring about thicker or thinner hair; things return to normal before long.

Sometimes the hormonal changes of the menopause or hereditary tendencies cause a thinning or receding at the front hairline and crown similar in pattern to traditional male baldness. Usually this indicates an over-sensitivity to the male hormones which occur in all humans. Hormone replacement therapy (HRT) often helps in these cases.

But hormones aren't always the culprit. A mysterious auto-immune disorder causes small, totally bald patches in the condition called *alopecia areata*. In most cases one or two bald spots appear, then regrow and all's well. In a few cases the hair loss continues, or the entire scalp hair or even all body hair falls out and stops growing. Stress or illness may trigger the disorder; medical research still seeks definitive causes.

Alas, there is no sure cure for hair loss, and GPs are sometimes unsympathetic, saying it doesn't hurt and it doesn't kill you. The GP is your first stop, however, for checks on blood iron and thyroid levels, and approval to try zinc and vitamin B12 supplements – treatments in these areas have been proven to help. You may ask to be referred to a specialist doctor who may try treating the scalp to stimulate follicles. Minoxodil (sold over the counter by pharmacists), steroid creams and a special scalp irritant acid can stimulate regrowth.

Headlice

Headlice and their eggs (nits) seem dirty and embarrassing, but they're as common as the common cold. Lice actually like clean hair, so having them is not a sign of poor hygiene. An itchy head is the most noticeable symptom; check all the family regularly, especially at hairline behind the ears and at the neck and along partings. Look for the tiny 2-mm ($1/12$th-inch) grey bugs and the even tinier white eggs glued to the hair. A special shampoo or conditioner from the pharmacy deals with the situation easily.

HAIR WOES?

If home treatment doesn't help, or if you have other hair and scalp worries, turn to your pharmacist, doctor or hairdresser. Your hairdresser may recommend a trichologist who's had several years' training in hair and scalp disorders. For more on hair professionals, see Chapter 7.

— Do-it-yourself, no-hype haircare —

Trichologist's trick

A good shampoo feels good: a good scalp cleaning feels wonderful – and can help with dandruff and lifeless hair. First, brew up a scalp tonic. Into a bowl pour 120 ml (4 fl oz) boiling water over one tablespoonful each of rosemary and sage or thyme. Let this cool, then add 40 ml (1 fl oz) witch hazel. Working from crown to front, then sides and back, part your hair (dry) into 3-cm (1-inch) rows and apply the tonic with cotton wool to your scalp. Shampoo and condition as usual. This takes a bit of time, but it's worth it for the heady, clear, wide-awake feeling.

Deep conditioning

Almond oil, coconut oil or fine olive oil gives dry, porous, dull hair new life and shine. Put three tablespoonfuls of the oil in a cup in a bowl of hot water to warm the oil. Warm a towel. Apply the warm oil to your dry hair. Massage into the hair, but avoid the scalp if your scalp is oily. Cover your hair with cling film or foil, then wrap the warm towel over the top and leave for 10 to 20 minutes. The heat helps the oil penetrate the cuticle. Shampoo and condition as usual.

Shiny rinse for normal and oily hair

A simple, healthy acid rinse closes hair cuticles extra-tight for super shine. After shampoo and rinsing, add two tablespoonfuls of vinegar or lemon juice to a cup of water and rinse through hair – don't rinse out.

Like taking shampoo from a baby

It's not home made, because some things are best left to experts, but baby shampoo is a minimalist's sure thing: uncomplicated, inexpensive, mild and perfectly satisfactory.

Hair alive

Any exercises that stimulate whole-body circulation (think aerobic) and any like the lion and shoulder stand (see 'Making faces' Chapter 4) that work on upper body and head microcirculation will help you to a healthy, growing headful of hair. Remember, it's the hair follicles in the scalp that need the cell-level conveyor belt of nutrients in, rubbish out. Two additional actions – easy and de-stressing – will also promote healthy hair via scalp microcirculation. (Don't do either of these if you have an oily scalp, for fear of stimulating even more oil production.)

A brush with destiny

Just before shampooing (or every day, if your hair condition is dry), bend over at the waist, hang your head down and brush your hair in long, vigorous strokes. This brings the blood to the scalp (healthy growth) and spreads oil from the scalp along the hair (shine, protection) and loosens any flakes of scalp skin. Follow each brush stroke with your other hand, smoothing the hair, to reduce static electricity.

Magic fingers

At any time, or when your conditioner is soaking in at hair-washing time, use your fingers to give your scalp a massage. Press your finger tips against the scalp and rotate the skin – it is naturally mobile. Start at the front hairline and work towards the nape. The stimulation brings blood and warmth to the scalp for health, growth – and tension release.

LIVING FOR HAIR

- Drink lots of water.
- Eat correctly. Protein (fish, poultry); fresh fruit and vegetables with every meal and for snacks; as little sugar and animal fat as possible.
- The hair vitamins and minerals are: A, B complex, sulphur, silicon, iodine, iron.
- Exercise, to stimulate scalp circulation.
- Shampoo regularly and always condition after shampoo.
- Use the right product for your hair needs.
- Have regular haircuts to trim off old ends.
- See Chapter 7 for style, curl and colour adventures with your hairdresser.

6

ESSENTIAL YOU: DEVELOPING PERSONAL STYLE

Everyone has style – it may be no-style or stand-out style or 100 per cent style. Style consists of clothes, accessories, hairstyle, make-up and most of all you. The development of your own personal style is a matter of strength versus confusion, confidence versus compliance, choice versus indecision. The best way to discover and polish your style is to know your personality and to combine this personality factor with the realities of your physical strengths and colour season. Start your style quest with the last of these three ingredients.

Colour me 'me': what's your season?

Before you can buy a single new garment, choose a lipstick or decide whether or not to dye your hair, you need to know the colour family that suits you. All ethnic skin types – white, oriental, Asian, black – have complexion undertones of yellow, blue or red. Complexion, eye and hair colour give each individual a natural colour tonality. The shirts, tops, collars, coats, scarfs, hair colour and make-up you wear reflect subtly shaded light on to the face. In the wrong shades you look sallow, tired, dull-eyed, worn; wrinkles and pores show more, you may even look ill. In the right colours your complexion looks clear, eyes sparkle, hair gleams, you look rested, refreshed, relaxed, healthy.

So which colours suit you? You can wear a rainbow of colours, but the trick is to find the depth, clarity and warmth of tone that give you life and natural glow, instead of murdering you. You do this by discovering which of the four main natural colour groups is yours – they're often named after the seasons of the year. Personal colour consultancies abound (check small ads in fashion magazines and local media), and a session is an excellent investment. But you may prefer to do it yourself the way the experts do, with four season-revealing colour swatch tests. It'll take some preparation and time – why not share the effort and the fun by doing it with a friend or two? The extra eyes and opinions help the process, too. Here's how ...

Prepare your colour test

1 Gather a selection of 18 to 35 plain coloured materials (now you see why it's easier to do this with a friend). Use sweaters, scarfs, jackets; borrow from the family; even use fabric or bath towels. Aim to collect:
   - the spectrum of the colour wheel: red, orange, yellow, green, blue, violet, ideally with two or more variations of each colour
   - the neutrals: black, grey, pure white, cream, browns, navy
   - sparkly lamé or sequin material in both gold and silver.
2 Gather up all the lipstick colour variations you can find.
3 Arrange the material colours on your bed or the floor, reds together, greens together, etc.
4 Strip your face of make-up and pull your hair back. Sit or stand in front of a mirror in good daylight. At each of the three colour tests you'll narrow down your season probabilities. By the end, you'll know which season you are.

First colour test: cool or warm?

Warm colours have a tinge of yellow, orange, red in them. Cool colours have a blue or green tinge. Many colours (pink, for instance) can be cool *or* warm, depending on the tone (for instance, sherbet blue-pink or strawberry warm pink).

Begin with the sparkly cloth, if you have it. Drape the gold around your neck and look at your face in the mirror. Now swap it for the silver. Gold is warm, silver is cool. Which makes you look drab, tired; which makes you look brighter, fresh?

Next (or instead) try a warm colour (say peach, orange, red, russet) around your neck. Then try a cool colour (such as sky blue, emerald, cobalt). Assess the effect on you. It won't always be easy; let your eyes attune themselves. Start making piles of 'yes', 'no', 'maybe' swatches ... a pattern begins to emerge.

Finally, if the 'yes' pile is mostly cool-toned, yours is a cool 'season': either winter or summer. If your 'yesses' are mostly warm, you are spring or autumn.

Second colour test: strong or soft?

What depth of colour suits you? What neutral? Swathe neck and shoulders in black and gaze at yourself. Now swap it for pure white. Which makes you look rested, alert? Which makes you look drained, strained?

If black is the one that enhances you, then black and dark, deep, saturated shades do most for you. You are a winter, maybe autumn, possibly spring.

If black kills you off, you'll find medium and pastel shades bring you to life. You are a summer or spring.

Now try the cream versus white, grey versus black, and try browns (cool and warm) and navy (cool). Which neutral suits you?

Third colour test: clear or muted?

What colour intensity suits you? Work through your 'yes' and 'maybe' piles of colour. If subtle, sludgy, dusty tones (for example mauve, olive, slate-blue) make you look elegant and relaxed, you are a mellow summer or autumn. If clear, sharp tones (like hot pink, acid yellow, turquoise) make you sparkle, you are a dramatic spring or winter.

Fourth colour test: lipstick confirmation

Finally, now feeling quite sure of your season, try on several lipsticks, using cleansing lotion to wipe away between tries. Which wash you out or overwhelm you? Which liven your complexion and eyes? Warm corals and peaches? Pinks – warm yellow-pinks or cool blue-pinks? Browns? Blue-red or orange-red or true red? This stage confirms your season.

ESSENTIAL YOU: DEVELOPING PERSONAL STYLE

Your season choices

Knowing your season does not mean you are forever wedded to periwinkle blue. Just about any colour can be worn by any season, so long as the shading variations are right. A sketchy scheme of the seasons' palettes follows here. Don't worry if you adore terracotta even though it's personal poison on you; you can still wear it – just not near your face. There are no hard-and-fast rules: let your own eyes and assessment make the final decisions.

Summer – a refined palette

Skin may be: ivory, pink beige, soft olive.
Some good colours: pewter, rose, amethyst, mauve, jade, true blue, pale yellow.
Good neutrals: grey, off-white.
Not-so-good colours: black, bright yellow, gold, yellow-green.

Autumn – an earthy palette

Skin may be: light, warm or golden brown, warm beige, bronze, ivory.
Some good colours: khaki, mahogany, rust, coral, mustard, moss, bronze, purple, turquoise.
Good neutrals: warm beige, chocolate brown.
Not-so-good colours: pure white, pastel pink, blue-red.

Winter – a striking palette

Skin may be: ivory, beige, clear olive, cool brown, black-brown.
Some good colours: hot pink, royal blue, fuchsia, blue-red, aubergine.
Good neutrals: black, white, navy.
Not-so-good colours: coral, orange, peach, brown.

Spring – a fresh palette

Skin may be: ivory, porcelain, beige, light olive.
Some good colours: salmon, tomato red, sky blue, bright blue, lemon.
Good neutrals: camel, ivory, milk chocolate.
Not-so-good colours: lavenders, blue-red, burgundy.

Style tips on body types

The big bonus: style has little to do with beautiful looks. In fact, being plain or having unusual features can be a definite advantage. Your own physical reality is a key factor in developing your personal style, for whatever your flaws and gems, you can make use of the visual laws of design to your style advantage. You surveyed your body basics in Chapter 1, now you need to make a closer assessment with style in mind. Have no fear, it's all good stuff.

Ten-step self assessment: the good, the bad, the good-enough

You may think you know everything about yourself. But do you? To check, stand before a full-length mirror, or even better a dressing-room three-way mirror. Sit and stand to observe. A measuring tape and a friend's second opinion will be a great help. Don't worry if you seem a disaster; it's how you are put together that matters, and discovering the gems that are the cornerstones of your style. Circle as many of the descriptions below that apply to you. If you have difficulty seeing yourself objectively, practise (secretly) assessing others, to develop your eye.

Step 1   Face shape

rounded, angular, long, oval.

Step 2   Neck

short, medium, long;
slender, medium, sturdy.

Step 3   Wrists and hands

small, medium, large;
lean, neat, stubby.

Step 4   Ankles and feet

small, medium, large;
neat, thick, wide.

ESSENTIAL YOU: DEVELOPING PERSONAL STYLE

Step 5 Bust

small, medium, large.

Step 6 Calculate head proportion

Measured head length (length from a book/straight edge on top of head to tip of chin):_____

Multiply head length x 8 = _____.

This is the height you should be if your head is in perfect balance. A smaller answer means your head proportion is small for your size; a larger answer means your head proportion is large (like many actresses and actors). Extremes demand careful attention to hair style.

Step 7 Calculate torso shape and proportion

Measure shoulder width and hips at widest points:

Shoulders _____ Hips _____

Shoulders wider than hips = broad shoulders.
Hips wider than shoulders = narrow shoulders.
Shoulders and hips same width = in balance.

To make the most of the best of you and to choose clothes to distract from the less-than-wonderful, taking shoulders, bust, midriff, waist, hips, stomach, thighs and bottom into account, decide whether your shape is mainly:

- straight – little waist definition
- curvy – some waist definition
- hourglass – good waist definition
- top heavy – broader or fuller on top than below the waist
- bottom heavy – broader or fuller below the waist than on top (pear-shaped)
- round – full on top and below waist, full stomach (apple-shaped)
- thick – wide waist and midriff and full above and below waist (barrel-shaped)?

Step 8 Calculate leg proportion

Measured leg length from widest point of hips to floor:_____

Subtract 2.5 cm (1 inch) from leg length, multiply by 2 = _____.

This is the height you should be for legs in perfect balance. A larger answer means your legs are long for your height (generally an advantage); a smaller answer means your legs are short for your height (help at hand from jacket and skirt length, waist and leg tricks).

Step 9   Study your current image

Put on your favourite outfit, one you feel good in, confident in. Study yourself carefully in the mirror. Why does it work for you? What does it do? Is it the colour? The length? The basic cut or design? Does it camouflage something you perceive as a problem (say big hips or thick waist)? Does it call attention to assets (say good legs, nice bust)?

Go through snapshots and videos of yourself – which clothes are best on you, which are mistakes? Why?

Step 10   Search out the gems

Feel like putting a tent over your body and a bag over your head? Stop. No one, not even the woman you regard as beautiful, is ever totally happy with her looks. The aim here is good-enough looks and polishing your gems. If there are negatives you can't or won't change (height? big stomach?) you can work around them, either by camouflage or by outshining them with emphasis on what you do like (good legs? great hair?). Much about looks is neutral. The short woman may wish she were tall, the tall woman wish she were short, some straight-haired women want perms, and some curly-heads want to iron their hair. With true personal style, anything goes; your attitude and a few tricks can make everything fine.

The visual laws of design dynamics

These four visual laws apply to paintings, architecture, package design, interiors, gardens ... and fashion, hair style, make-up and you. They are the facts of how the human eye works.

Law of lines: Vertical lines lengthen and narrow the way something looks. Horizontal lines widen and broaden. Diagonal lines direct, distract or excite.

Law of colours: Dark fades things away, distances, makes things appear smaller. Light brings forward, enlarges.

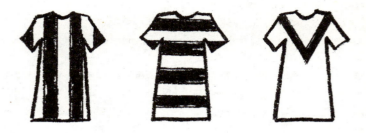

Figure 6 Visual laws of design dynamics

Law of detail: Busy-ness attracts the eye. Simplicity soothes, blanks out.

Golden rule of style: Style-wise, in clothes, make-up and hair, you can use the laws as you wish. Probably you would like to avoid looking fat, stumpy, gawky or scrawny. If so, combine the three laws into one golden rule: *Don't use line, colour or detail to emphasise a part of yourself you don't like.*

Strategic dressing

Some dressing choices will generally flatter you. Some will exaggerate the things you'd rather hide. Some will spotlight your assets, a double plus for making you shine and for distracting attention from parts you'd rather leave in the dark. The secret of personal style is the development of an instinct for choosing cut, colour, pattern, fabric and detail that work for you.

Attention distractors: downplay body exaggerations

Broad shoulders, big on top: try longline jackets, V-neck, scoop-neck, raglan sleeves. Avoid shoulder pads.

Narrow shoulders: try loose tops, boat necklines, padded shoulders, scarf or brooch worn to upper right or left.

Full bust: try soft, loose jackets, small patterns, scoop neck, V-neck, draped neck. Avoid short sleeves, cropped waist tops, details.

Small bust: try loose, easy fits on top, details. Avoid clingy fabrics.

Thick waist: try loose, long or boxy jackets, long tops, tunics, blousons. Avoid contrasting belts.

Rounded stomach: try soft-pleated, A-line or flared skirts, soft-pleated trousers, broad shoulder lines, darker, unpatterned bottoms. Avoid centre buttons and details.

Flat bottom: try unconstructed jackets that end below your bottom, chemise or drop-waist dresses. Avoid clingy fabrics.

Short or thick legs: try dark hose or hose to match dress; skirt at or just below knee, or long; trousers; boots; moderate heels. Avoid contrasting colours below the knee.

Attention getters: call the eye to your assets

Good bust and midriff: try fitted dresses, and tops, clingy fabrics.

Nice waist and hips: try waisted jackets, contrast-colour belts, wide belts, fitted dresses, slim skirts.

Great legs: try flesh-coloured hose, shorter skirts, leggings, good and interesting shoes.

Good complexion: try scoop- and V-necks, jewellery and detail near the face.

Good hands: try rings, bracelets, three-quarter length sleeves.

Undercover story

A well-fitting bra helps your bust keep its shape or improve it, and makes your clothes hang well. A bra bought at a department store usually costs the same as an over-the-counter one, with the bonus of being able to try it on and often being advised by experienced, trained fitters. Slips give a smoother line to skirts. Be sure knickers (always with cotton crotch to avoid thrush) don't show up as a panty line with tight trousers or clingy fabrics. Consider stretchy control panties to firm flab (and/or get going on your exercises!).

Jacket to the rescue

A jacket (or two or three) can pull outfits together, look right for nearly any occasion, and solve a myriad of negatives, depending on the jacket.

- *Long jackets* (to below your bottom), whether loose fitting or boxy, hide fullness of waist, hip, bottom, bust, midriff.
- *Crop-waist jackets* compliment short women, good waists and hips.
- *Unstructured, easy uncluttered jackets* unify short women, heavy women.
- *Fitted jackets* show off slim waists.
- *Double-breasted jackets* or layered jacket-sweater-shirt add bulk to thin figures.
- *Blazers* go with jeans and skirts and trousers.

Accessories with attitude

Whatever the items, accessories can work wonders. They can pull an outfit together. They can be strategic ploys (see 'Attention-getters' and '-distractors', too), and they can be style beacons (if they are talking points or personality spotlights).

- *Belts*, wide and contrast-coloured, spotlight a good waist. Belt buckles can draw interest. Belts that are narrow and the same colour as clothes minimise middle-body flaws.
- *Brooches*, centred they accentuate the vertical. To one side they create diagonal interest.
- *Necklaces* and *earrings* provide top interest. Shorter, rounded ones soften, long ones add vertical lines. Pearls give soft light to the face.
- *Scarves* add dashes of colour to neutrals, or allow 'poison' colours you love but can't normally wear. They draw attention to face and neck. Hung long, they add vertical lines to distract from wideness. Knotted to one side they soften.

Style directions: attitude in action

The height of style – your personal style – is the look in which you feel at ease and in command of yourself. True style is based on force of personality – today's word for it is 'attitude'. Starting with the following four cardinal style points, which feels most like you? (Wishful or actual.)

- Classic – tailored, elegant, calm.
- Natural – easy, sportive, relaxed.
- Creative – dramatic, bold, energetic.
- Soft – flowing, gentle, sensual.

If you instinctively are drawn to one of the four directions, or to a variation (name it yourself!), does your present style project this? Could it be heightened?

STYLE WARS – BUT ...!

- I'm classic *and* creative!
- I'm short and have great legs!
- I'm busty but flat-bottomed!
- I'm an autumn but I hate terracotta!
- I hate rules about anything!

These lists and tips don't mean you have to wear these designs, and don't mean you can't wear others. Watch for what works on someone whose assets or drawbacks are similar to yours. Watch for what works on you and look to buy more of it. When you shop, pick out some things you might not normally try, see how they look.

You can throw the design guidelines out of the window if they don't suit your personal style direction; it's up to you. You might even want to ...

Turn a lemon into lemonade

The 100 per cent stylist may look at her 'flaws' and decide to flaunt them. Playing up the extraordinary takes courage, but can give great confidence; it's 'in your face' attitude. A certain amount of self-mockery helps to carry this off, though this does not mean bad-mouthing yourself. Some examples:

- *Big nose*: Sleek hair back, wear big earrings, exotic turbans and clothes. Or go for an austere, nun-like look or ethnic strength. Forget pretty; be bold.
- *Big mouth*: Make the most of it with bright red, pink or orange lipstick. Laugh and smile, pout and pose. Dark glasses will make your mouth the focus.
- *Small, stubby hands*: Don't hide them. Cover them in rings galore, the more the better. Wear intense nail polish. Jangle chunky bangle bracelets. Gesticulate as you talk.

- *Overweight*: Blossom, be proud, big. Wear bold, bright colours and patterns, startling jewellery, big hat, big hair.

Thin, freckled, tall, tiny, whatever you are, break some of the rules and make your mark as being *you*.

Consider a trademark

If you feel more comfortable being a mild to moderate stand-out, think about the colours, personality direction, designs that are the essential you, and add or develop a 'something' that is always particularly you. It could be...

- *Colour, fabric:* Always black and red. Or always tans. Or always knits, or solids. Less is usually more, when it comes to style.
- *A sort of uniform:* T-shirt and trousers. Suit. Or never-in-trousers. Or long skirts.
- *Antique jewellery:* Or ethnic jewellery. Or crafted-by-you jewellery. Build a collection.
- *Always a long necklace:* Or pearls. Or bracelets or rings or dangly earrings.

Ages and stages of style

The younger you are, the more likely you are to get caught up by trendy fashion. That's great (so long as it isn't a body-shape disaster): after all, you're the wave of the future, the cutting edge of what's new, and your role in life is to be different from the older generation.

Into your *twenties, thirties and forties,* work responsibilities may demand new, more serious style directions. Your growing maturity (and income, perhaps) makes this a good time to develop your personal sense of style. Motherhood may cramp your style, but remember that the right-coloured jumper and lipstick can lift you during the shapeless, sleepless-nights stage; later, a dash of style can rescue you from the practicalities of the jeans/leggings/sweatpants doldrums.

In your *forties* and especially in your *fifties and beyond*, you have the chance to let your style flourish. You're older, wiser, more confident than before, free to refine and emphasise your personal style. As gravity and biology have their way with you, style is the counterforce – go for it.

As you get older, your natural hair and skin tones may subtly change; black, say, or muted colours, may become draining and add unnecessary years to your looks. Run a season recheck now and then. You may need to adjust with lighter or darker, clearer or subtler shades.

Don't, above all, as you get into your *seventies and beyond*, settle for safe saggy dresses and crimped little perms; keep your style banner flying.

Your own before-into-after style plan

Based on your self-assessments, you've now got several parameters to juggle when it comes to polishing your personal style. You've discovered what colours flatter you, what physical assets you want to spotlight, what flaws you want to de-emphasise, how the visual laws of design work. You have a feeling for the personality direction that puts you in control. Now it's time to see your style in action.

Five-step wardrobe weedout and build-up

You can pay a wardrobe consultant to do this for you. It'll cost at least two weeks' salary and it can be a brilliant investment (some shops and colour consultancies offer the service, or look for small ads in fashion magazines). But you can do it yourself. The main ingredient is a clutch of plastic, rubbish-bin bags.

Step 1

Go through every item of clothing you own. If you haven't worn it in two or three years, put it in a bag.

Step 2

Try on everything else. Is it in your season, does the colour flatter? If not, but you love it anyway, can you add a scarf or other top interest to counter the effect? How about fit, fabric and the visual laws of verticals and horizontals, light and dark, detail and simplicity? What works, really works for your physical realities and your personality? What's so-so? Put disasters and so-sos into a bin bag.

Step 3

Go through shoes and jewellery, scarfs and belts with the same ruthless intent. Style is spare and focussed, not waffly.

Step 4

Take the bin bags of clothes to your favourite charity shop. If this pace is too fast for you, put them in the attic; if you don't miss the items for a year, bite the bullet and then take them to the charity shop. It will feel good to let go. If even this is too drastic, you can simply think your way through your wardrobe, mentally assessing your clothes as you ease into your personal style; eventually you'll do your weedout.

Step 5

So now what? Maybe you've pared your wardrobe down to only six outfits – that's fine: style is less, style is intent. Should you race out and spend bundles on new clothes? No: even if you can afford it, too much all at once can mean mistakes. Start by buying one or two just-right-for-you essentials: a sweater or dress, a jacket or suit, trousers or a skirt. Perhaps a brooch or necklace. The aim is slowly to build your look as you grow into your own personal style.

Fighting the fashion minefield

Some people love to shop, some hate it. Either way, it's easy to lose your sense of personal style among racks of clothes. Fashion is a major distractor, for fashion is not style. Learn to laugh at the changes of colours that come and go every season; use them, don't let them use you. Waists up, waists down, polka dots out, florals in? It's easy to be persuaded – and, face it, sometimes you just want something trendy and fun. But double-check how it looks on you. And if it's bound to be a passing fad, don't spend a lot. Stick to your flattering shades, even if it means no new clothes this spring (if you have to buy, your neutrals will always be around somewhere). Hold tight to your own style, triumph over the marketeers and the lemmings; be you.

Notice that I haven't mentioned money or designer clothes yet. Name labels may be better made, of better fabrics than cheap things – but they are no guarantee of style. In fact, they may throw you off your style, making you choose something that has the wrong lines or something that's too safe, just because of the name and the price tag. If you can afford top quality or designer clothes, aim for basics, because they'll last for years. Style-wise you can do quite well with moderately priced clothes. Cheap, street-market clothes can also provide style, although they won't be well tailored or hard wearing. Smart, financially pressed shoppers can find real bargains in good-as-new and charity shops.

I suggest a little meditation session before you hit the stores – visualise the clothes you own that work for you, visualise your colours, see yourself and the purpose of your expedition (a dress for a wedding? some summer shorts and tops?). Don't fix too firm a goal – successful shopping is an almost mystic state of being focussed yet open: on track, fully aware of your style and your needs, yet alert to inspiration, to serendipity. Buy the right thing when you see it; it may not pass your way again.

Finally, if you really love something, buy it. Even if it's 'wrong', if you love it, you'll wear it with flair and confidence which is the essence of style. And when you do make wardrobe mistakes, try to learn from them – what fooled you into thinking those jeans fit well? What convinced you to buy that mustard jumper?

Other distractions from personal style

Work ethic. The required or unspoken uniform for your place and kind of work is sometimes necessary, but sometimes the pressue to fit in brainwashes you into following a not-you style.

Social pressures. Dressing to be in with, or to out-do, friends, family and people around you may steer you into clothes, hair, make-up that diminish the best of you.

Husband or partner. Loves you with long hair, hates women in long/short skirts, thinks trousers are only for casual times, can't stand any sort of change ….

Sales and bargains. The price blinds you to the fact that it's the wrong colour, too long, doesn't go with anything … .

If you recognise any of these these personal style side-tracking tendencies in yourself, it's a sure sign that you need to develop more sense of self in your image. Just like diet, exercise, hair and make-up before-into-afters, you need to make changes slowly, so that those around you don't inhibit you, and – very important – so that you feel fully confident as the emerging new you. Here are some personal style-sense beginnings ...

Nine ways to develop your personal style

1 *Be a style spy*. There's someone in your immediate life whose look and flair you admire. How does she do it, what is her style? There are lots of others who have no particular style. What could they do better? Look at strangers in the shops, on your journey to work; mentally style them, develop your style eye.
2 *Develop your outlook and attitude*. Collect quotes and sayings and put them on your wall, around your mirror, on your fridge, in a notebook. Get them from newspapers and magazines, greeting cards, books, TV, radio, songs, books of quotes. What confirms you, cheers you, motivates, defines you?
3 *Ignore, generally, the fashion models on the catwalk and the glossy pages*. They aren't real people in the real world; their style isn't their own. It is carefully concocted by designer, editor, stylist, make-up artist, photographer. However, you can adapt some ideas from these dream images, and from rock and film stars and other celebrities, too.
4 *Keep a journal or diary*. For a week, at the end of each day, write down everything you did in the day, hour by hour. Then, or after the week is up, write why you did each thing. This will define your priorities and pressures. It can confirm your chosen direction, and may reveal areas you'd like to rethink. True style is individuality, finding your own path, sticking to it, growing with it.
5 *Steal ideas and role models from history books and art museums*. Queen Alexandra wore huge chokers and curls on her forehead, Dutch beauties pulled their hair straight back off their foreheads, Elizabeth I flaunted her long, elegant fingers, Isadora Duncan wore loose flowing robes, Marilyn Monroe had a rounded stomach. Today's beauty and fashion looks limit you to today's ideas of admirable bodies and clothes, but your body and personal style may not conform. Look further afield for inspiration and originality.
6 *Play the party game, 'If I were a car I'd be a ...'*. Go through lots of categories, do it with friends to see how you see each other. Going back to the four cardinal style personality directions, if you were a

fabric, would you be gaberdine (classic), denim (natural), taffeta (creative), chiffon (soft)? You disagree with these identifications? Good! Define your own – style is everything to do with attitude.

7 *Work on your voice and speech.* Practise reading or talking into a tape recorder. Choose something from a newspaper or magazine, maybe leave your tape on as you talk on the phone. Play back and listen. Is your voice hesitant, wispy, apologetic, full of 'errs' and 'ums'? Is it vibrant, lively, commanding? Practise to improve, using your tape recorder. To prepare for presentations or interviews, ask a friend to video you.

8 *Work on your movement and posture.* If your body self-assessment revealed awkwardness, take action. Yoga, dance class, Alexander Technique or home exercises can help (see Chapters 3 and 10). Moving and being still with deliberate grace creates a space around you, an air of conscious presence. That's style. (P.S. It helps clothes look good, too.)

9 *Practise rebellion.* Work on your anger, find your own path. Style is about not conforming, so even if you're a soft, romantic summer or a light, natural spring you don't have to follow rules about being proper and basically invisible. Discovering what makes you angry (in society, in family life, in work practice) can be a great fuel to energise your individual style. A defiant 'so there' may be an unusual brooch, a bright scarf, sexy underwear, an amazing pair of earrings, perfect shoes – a signal that you are *you*.

100 PER CENT STYLISTS OF THE 20TH CENTURY

Mae West – flaunted her sexuality and laughed with it, too. Utterly outrageous confidence, hair, make-up and (of course) body.

Katharine Hepburn – thoroughbred looks, tall, slim, impeccable bearing. A natural aristocrat in all circumstances. Made trousers an elegant must for women.

Diana Vreeland – as fashion editor of US *Vogue* in the 60s set style trends for millions. Turned her very plain looks into a unique daily uniform: lacquered black hair, alabaster skin, perfectly tailored black suit.

Quentin Crisp – artists' model and British author of *The Naked Civil Servant*, he defined himself and forged his style out of sheer willpower.

Style projection

Style file

Beyond clothes, hair, make-up and manner, style is a fact of your immediate environment. You can make your mark on your workplace desk, your car, your notebooks, your home. With your pens, your stationery, your food, your flowers, your parties. Via colour, design and force of personality you can establish your signature, own your territory, imprint your essential style.

Fragrance

The ultimate style projection, fragrance wafts before you as you enter a room, it surrounds your presence, it lingers after you leave. It can 'say' you are sensual or fresh or dynamic or old-fashioned or.... See Chapter 9 for tips on body chemistry and the art of selecting the fragrances that work best for you.

THE BEST STYLE SECRET

A man's white T-shirt is a never-go-wrong classic that you can dress up, dress down, wear under a business suit, with a skirt short or long, over a swimsuit, and naturally partner with jeans, or with trousers and jacket. Don't be without one (or six).

7

HAIR: YOUR MOST FLEXIBLE BEAUTY ASSET

Your best hairstyle is one that suits your face shape, your body proportions, your personal style and your hair's behaviour. A tall order! Hair is your most versatile good-looks asset. Of course, it's at its best when it is clean, shiny and healthy (see Chapter 5), but what style, what cut, and what about colour and curl?

Four-part self-assessment: what hairstyle for you?

Part 1 Your face shape

It can be surprisingly hard to know your own face shape. If you're not sure, get a ruler, pull your hair back from your face, and go to a mirror.

1 Measure the length of your face from hairline to chin.
2 Measure face width across the widest part, the cheekbones.

You can further define your face shape by holding two straight-edges vertically (rulers, pencils, combs) at the outer corners of your eyes. The area left outside the lines shows the width or narrowness of forehead, cheekbones, cheeks, jaw.

The secret of a flattering hairstyle is to find one that does not exaggerate any exaggerations you already have. Study yourself and figure it out.

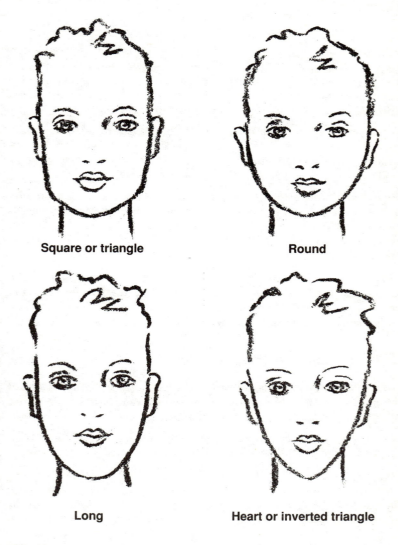

Figure 7 Face shapes

Oval: Face length is 1½ times the width. This is the ideally balanced face, not too soft, not angular. Any hairstyle will suit you; a simple, no-fringe, off-the-face one will show off your classic oval.

Round: The width nearly equals the length. A hairstyle with height at the crown helps to 'verticalise' (remember 'The visual laws of design dynamics', Chapter 6). Or try a centre parting or a geometric, angular cut to counteract the roundness. Short hair is often best. Generally, avoid curls that echo the curves of your face, or the straight-across fringe that focusses attention on plump, round cheeks.

Long: Face length is more than 1½ times the width. A curled or layered style with width at the sides of the face breaks up the impression of length. A low, side parting can also help. Avoid long, straight hair and centre partings; these just emphasise the vertical.

Square or triangle: A wide, strong jaw. A square shape has equally wide cheekbones and forehead; the triangle narrows toward cheekbones and forehead. Soften the angularity with waves, curls or feathery wisps. Avoid width at jaw or a blunt cut that ends right at the jaw.

Heart or inverted triangle: Wide at forehead, narrower at jaw and chin. The heart shape is softer, wider at the cheekbones than the more angular inverted triangle. Short or shoulder-length styles with a full crown downplay the upper width; avoid width at the cheekbones.

Part 2 Your body features

You 'wear' your hair and you wear your clothes, so the same visual design dynamics apply. As you think about your hairstyle, consider the overall balance and your body realities.

Very big or heavy: Some volume and length to hair will fit you best. Styles too wide or full, or very short and flat contrast sharply with the rest of you.

Very small: You can look terrific with very short hair, or add some height with short or medium-length styles that have some height at the crown. Avoid wide, full styles that threaten to turn you into a mushroom.

Very thin: Long, straight hair will only emphasise your vertical lines. Try short or medium styles with bounce, waves or curls.

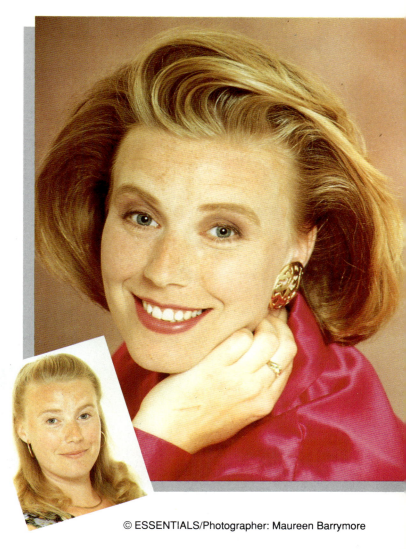

© ESSENTIALS/Photographer: Maureen Barrymore

How can new make-up, a new hairstyle and the right colours before-into-after you?
Start by assessing yourself – colour season, face shape, hair profile, style attitudes. This natural blonde has kept her hair all one length, but lifted it to a face-framing medium length with slight layering at the ends. Styling mousse and blow-drying give height at hair roots for an easy-going yet classic style. Her new make-up is classic, too, with a light foundation and a palette of rosy, plum-beige pinks for eyes and cheeks, soft brown for brows and lashes, and a dramatic blued-pink for lips. The strong, clear-toned blouse flatters her cool season.

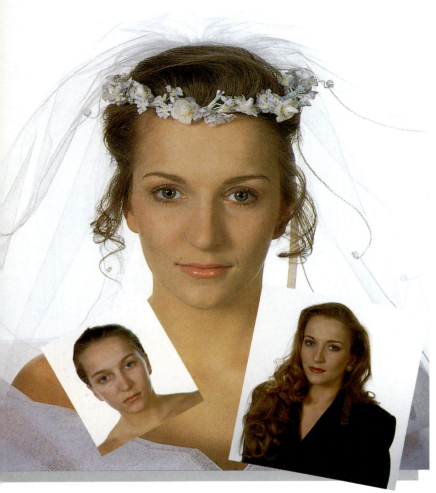

Here comes the... many faces of you
From bare-faced to full make-up, for different occasions. Both looks are created with 12 make-up steps, starting with foundation and powder, but they use different colours and subtleties of application. The out-to-impress evening make-up uses medium-dark grey eyeshadow, definitive eyeliner, warm blusher and glossy red lipcolour. After setting on hot rollers, her curls have been gently separated, not completely brushed through.

Wedding day for the classic bride calls for a lighter palette – using pale pink (or peach for autumns and springs) for the main eyeshadow, very thin smudged-down eyeliner, a soft glow of pink (or peach) blush, and pink-coral lipstick – carefully applied so it lasts as long as possible.

How to choose the right foundation

Whatever your complexion colour, the aim of foundation is to look like skin. The wrong shade can give you a chalky, orangey or brown mask-like look. Don't test a foundation on the back of your hand, it's darker and rougher than your face.

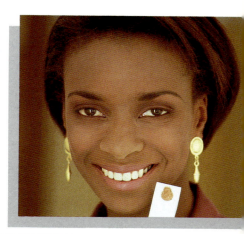

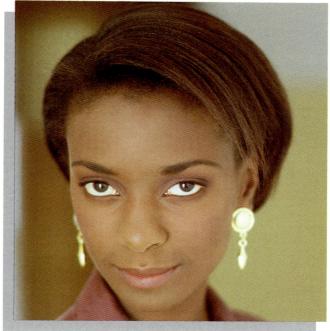

© ESSENTIALS/Photographer: Caroline Summers

Instead smooth it on your inside arm, just above the wrist, or on your neck. It should match your skin colour exactly, practically disappearing, except for the texture.

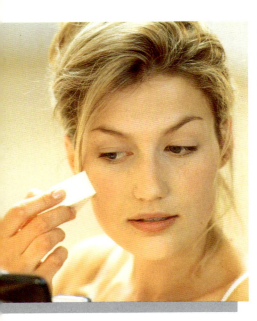

Step-by-step make-up
Whatever your personal style and whatever the occasion, you have a dozen make-up steps at your command (see pages 118–25). You can choose to be a minimalist and take only four steps, or be a subtle or definitive stylist at six to ten steps, or go all the way to achieve making-a-statement make-up.

Complexion steps
On freshly cleansed and moisturised skin, dot foundation on your forehead, then blend it up to the hairline and out to the temples. Use a damp sponge, as here, or your fingertips. Dab more foundation on one cheek and blend under the eye, then downwards and outwards. Repeat on the other side. Continue with nose, eyelids, browbone, then lip, chin and jawline. A powder-cream compact, shown here, requires no separate powder dusting.

© ESSENTIALS/Photographer: Paul Viant

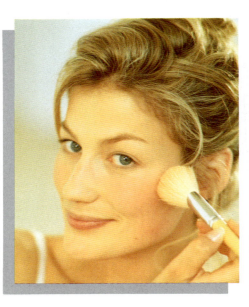

Powder blush is the easiest glow of colour to achieve, whether on bare skin or after foundation or powder. Start the colour in line with your pupil when looking straight ahead, and wing it up in a crescent towards the temple. Blend blush edges to a whisper.

Some people prefer to apply blush *after* eye make-up to ensure that the eyes hold the main focus of the face. Try both ways to see which order you prefer.

Eye steps

After tidying and defining brows (see pages 118–19 and 122), apply a light shade of eyeshadow all over the eyelid, working from inner towards outer corner. Use pencils, sponge-tip applicators or brushes – experiment to see which you prefer, aiming always for subtle blending, no harsh lines of colour. Here, a sponge-tip applies a lighter shade right up to the brow, where it serves as a highlighter. A brush feathers a darker shade along the eyelid crease and near lashes at the outer part of the eyes.

Eyeliner comes next, if desired. These slightly hooded eyes gain balance from a smudge of colour along bottom lashes from outer corner to centre. Here, darker shadow has been used instead of liner. Complete the eye emphasis with two coats of darkest brown mascara (allow to dry between coats), meticulously applied to top and bottom lashes.

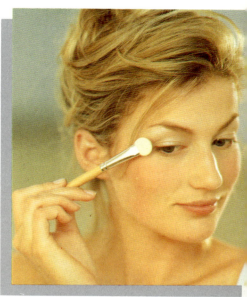

© ESSENTIALS/Photographer: Paul Viant

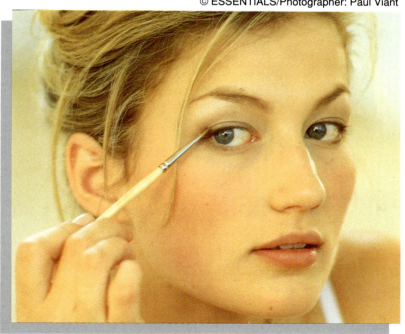

Lip steps

Lipcolour looks and lasts best if you start with lip pencil. Choose a shade close to your lipstick or to natural brown-red lipcolour. Simply draw from the centre to corners of top lip, then bottom lips. Soften the line slightly with a finger, as shown. For a natural, moist look, just apply lipgloss and you're done.

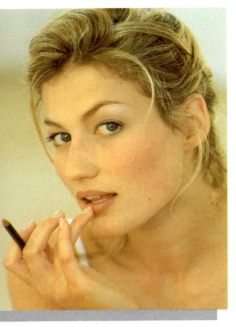

© ESSENTIALS/Photographer: Paul Viant

For colour and flair, nothing beats lipstick, and nothing betters the lasting-power and perfection of application by lipbrush. Paint on the colour – the lipliner stops colour 'bleeding' on to the skin around the lips.

This golden, spring season model has used eight make-up steps, and chosen a classic make-up palette of brown-beige shadows, browned-pink blush and coral-red lipcolour.

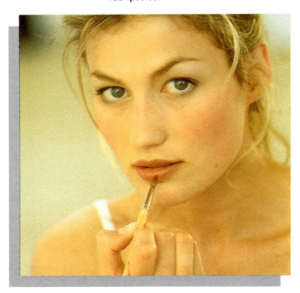

Subtle stylist

This cool, summer blonde has highlighted her naturally wavy hair and cut it to a medium-length, partly layered style to allow for its texture. Waves and curls soften her angular jaw. In six make-up steps she prefers to use no foundation or powder and to use eye make-up with a light hand, but she's not afraid to flaunt some glossy soft-red lipstick. The overall impact: casual, but with an eye for flair.

© ESSENTIALS/
Photographer: Nigel Limb

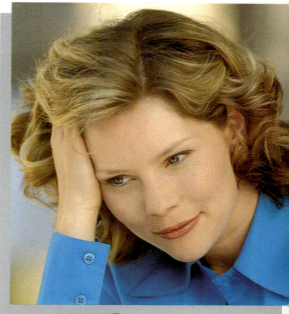

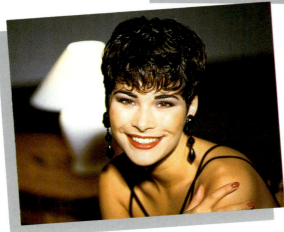

© ESSENTIALS/
Photographer:
David Levine

Making a statement

Here's one way to go from day into a high-profile night look, even if you can't get home to change. This dramatic winter brunette has gelled her short layered hair and tousled it into crisp curls. Black eyeliner and violet eyeshadows, high cheek colour and dazzling true red lipstick provide sparkle. To complete the picture: nails in matching true red, dangly earrings and an expanse of smooth, bare skin.

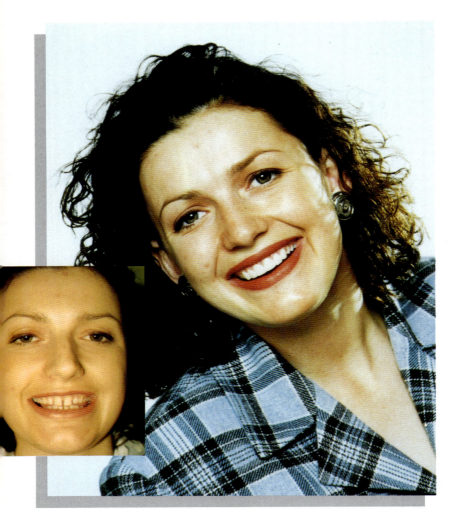

Smiles are beautiful

Perhaps the look of your teeth stops you from smiling as often as you could? Cosmetic dental improvements can be surprisingly easy and reasonably priced. Veneers – individually tailored from wafer-thin porcelain – can be permanently bonded on to your own teeth to cover up or fill in front-teeth flaws. The transformation of the gaps in this smile used six veneers, fitted and fixed in place in only two appointments. Some cosmetic corrections take only one visit, others require more time and expense – but the results can be dramatically worth it. See Chapter 11 for more information.

Dental correction by Dr Russell Craddock BDS. Dentics Cosmetic Dental Studios, King's Road, Chelsea, London.

Large nose or high shoulders: Avoid a full, straight fringe and Cleopatra-type blunt-cut. These squash down a face (fine for talls and thins) and focus attention just where you don't want it.

Deep-set eyes, low forehead, or small face: Keep hair off the face, with no overhanging fringe, to prevent eyes becoming pools of dark shadow.

Part 3 Your personal style

Essential you

Colour or high-fashion cuts will appeal to someone with creative, dramatic style. Waves, soft curls or wisps signal a sensualist. Practical, straight hair or casual softness say sportive. Bobs and simplicity are for classicists. Your hairstyle has got to be one you feel comfortable with, and it can project an effect of your choosing. You've also got to consider lifestyle – do you need a no-fuss, wash-and-wear style, does your work require trimly-groomed looks, do you have time to spend on a complicated hairstyle?

Style wars

So a geometric style would suit your rounded features, but your hair was born to curl? So you'd like to try a radical short cut even though you're big? So do what you most need to do? Explore your possibilities, but above all, be happy in your hair, even if it breaks the rules.

Ages and stages of hairstyles

As your years earn you lines and wrinkles it's usually best to soften a hairstyle, and, at some point, to let hair lighten to its natural grey or silver, complementing the change to a thinner-skinned complexion. But don't be brainwashed into a sensible perm or short cut; let your hair suggest what to do – on an over-60 year old, French-twisted white hair or a shining straight cap of silver can look striking.

Part 4 Your hair's behaviour

Hair has a mind of its own, and its behaviour – thin, flyaway, lank, thick, wildly wavy, etc. (see Chapter 5, too) – certainly affects your choice of hairstyle. You can explore cuts and styles that make the most of what you've got. Or with cut, styling products and tools, colour and perms you can coax and control your hair. After you've self-assessed your hairstyle options, gleaned hairstyle ideas from magazine pages (here's the time when it *is* useful to look at models) and from people you see in everyday life, your hairdresser holds the key to managing your willful head of hair.

— To the hairdresser: the cut is all —

Word of mouth is the best way to find a good hairdresser; if you like a friend's haircut, ask who did it. Otherwise, just keep trying likely-looking salons until you hit gold. When you find a hairdresser who pleases you, treasure her or him! Not all will have the same knack with your particular hair and your personality. To get the style you want, it helps to know the terminology.

Style options: how to talk to your hairdresser

One-length cut A basic hair shape of all one length. Straight or bob style may be **taper cut** (also called **slither** or **feather cut**) subtly to thin and shape the ends. **Blunt cut** (sometimes called **precision** or **club cut**) keeps all ends at one length; makes hair look heavy and thick, good for thin or fine hair.

Layered cut Hair is carefully cut at slightly different lengths to make hair lie smoother or to show off curls or waves. Long or medium-length hair can be a basic one-length cut with slight layering at the ends to encourage it to turn under, curve up or curl. Or short, medium or long hair can be layered all over, for lots of curl and movement.

Graduated cut Exaggerated layers or steps of hair length. May be **short graduation** – longish on top and clipped below in a sort of Norman soldier look, good on shiny sleek hair. **Long graduation,** also called **long layered cut** – means shorter lengths on top of head blend into layers of medium or long hair; this suits thick or wavy and curly hair.

Front line of style Cut of your hair across the forehead and hairline; face shape affects your choice. It might be straight ('Cleopatra' fringe), arc (soft curls or fringe framing face), asymetrical (side parting, hair an upside-down V on forehead), etc. Hair can also be waved or pulled straight back from forehead.

HAIR: YOUR MOST FLEXIBLE BEAUTY ASSET

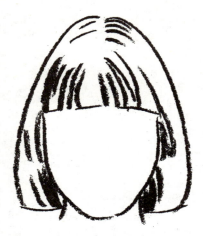

One-length cut with straight front line

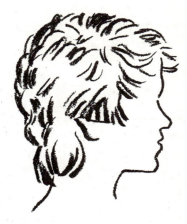

Layered cut (short) with arc front line, stepped side line

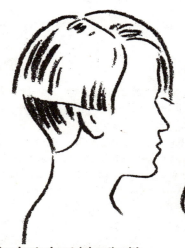

Graduated cut (short) with V front line, stepped side line, curved nape

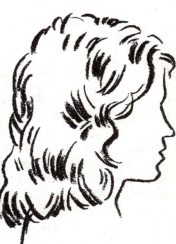

Graduated cut (long), with arc front line, diagonal side line, V back line

Figure 8 Hair talk

Side line of style Cut of your hair in profile; body proportions should be taken into consideration. Options include horizontal (one length at earlobes, chin or longer), stepped (shortish hair horizontal at ear, then shaped to nape), diagonal (hair slants shorter at front, longer towards back), reverse diagonal.

Back line of style You need two mirrors to see this; assess neck, body proportions and hair behaviour. Medium or long hair can hang as a horizontal, rainbow arc, or 'smile' arc. Short hair can show the nape as a V, W, or soft curve. Hair might also be plaited, French pleated, swept up.

Natural parting Your hairdresser should comb your clean, wet hair straight back off your face, and then gently push at the crown. The hair parts naturally, revealing its in-born growth pattern. Heed it; your style will last much longer if it follows its natural fall.

Movement Also called **texture**, this means the hair is cut or styled to show off waves or curls. Movement can also describe the way that precision-layered, straight hair swings into place.

Definition Mousse, gel or other styling product emphasises curls or ends of hair, giving crispness instead of leaving them a soft mass.

Tame Calming thick, curly, wavy, frizzy or flyaway hair through a cut or styling products.

Volume Bulk or thickness of hairstyle. Cut, perm or colouring can give volume if you don't have it naturally.

Lift Height at the roots. Blow-dry, root-perm, set or backcombing can provide lift.

Afro hair Natural, tight Afro curls should be lifted and shaped with a wide-toothed hair pick, and cut when hair is dry for a perfect shape and even balance. Or hair can be pressed or permed, then cut and styled in any way. Intricate corn rows, plaits, hair weaving and extensions or wild dreadlocks are further options.

Keep talking to your hairdresser

Tousled, **soft**, **casual** is the opposite of **smooth**, **sleek** or **geometric**. Then there's **wild**, full hair and **scrunched** curls. Or a **firm hold** style. Or a **spiky** look. Or hair with **bounce**. Or ... the words and the looks will keep on changing. Stay *au courant* by reading beauty and fashion magazines. For a new hairstyle, or a reshaping of your present one, do take along magazine pictures or snapshots of yourself – but listen to your hairdresser's advice as to whether your chosen style will be successful with your hair health, texture, thickness and with your face shape and body proportions. On the other hand, don't let her or him talk you into a style that's not essentially you (review 'Style directions', 'Fighting the fashion minefield' and 'Nine ways to develop your personal style' in Chapter 6). Be sure, too, to ask about upkeep of a style you have doubts about, and how to style your hair at home.

Above all, if you're not getting what you want, speak up; your hairdresser can't read your mind and does want you to be happy.

Hair grows at a rate of about 1.25 cm ($^{1}/_{2}$ inch) per month, and it grows at different rates in different places on your head ... so to keep your hair from getting shaggy and shapeless you need to see your hairdresser every four to eight weeks.

Regular cuts are also vital to keep hair healthy. All 'old' hair tends to split at the ends; cutting is the only cure. See Chapter 5 for more on hair health.

Styling at home

The cut is all, but now you're on your own. The right equipment, products and a few inside secrets will help you master the art of styling your hair yourself.

Tooling-up for home hairstyling

- **Vent brush** has holes in its base, for quicker drying of casual, tousled styles.
- **Circular or radial brush** stretches and shapes hair into curls – choose smaller diameter for tighter curls, larger for looser or for the ends of long hair. It can tangle hair easily, so go slowly and carefully.
- **Flat brush** allows smooth hair to be pulled straight, and possibly to have a slight curve under or up at the ends.
- **Straight comb** for parting hair to dry or set it section by section. You need a **wide-toothed comb** (also called rake comb) for wet hair.

- **Hair pick** (Afro comb) for Afro hair and many others. Use it to lift and arrange curls of naturally dried or blow-dried, scrunched hair because brushing through would create mere waves or even frizz.
- **Sectioning clips** to hold other sections of hair out of the way as you deal with one section.
- **Rollers and clips** of various sizes for tighter or looser curls and lift, if you prefer this method.
- **Blow drier** with varied speed and heat settings plus a nozzle for concentrated airflow to roots, curls or length of hair. And/or a diffuser for gentle air on scrunched, layered, curly styles.
- **Crimping iron** gives tiny waves, an angel-hair effect with thickness and volume.
- **Electric tongs, hot brush, hot rollers** to use after blow dry or between shampoos to firm the shape of curls or waves.
- **Hood drier** gives general all-over heat for hair set on rollers. More used in salons than at home these days.

Product lowdown: styling aids before drying

Blow-dry lotion, **mousse**, **sculpting gel**, **moulding mist**, **serum**... These miracle workers coat hair with a very fine film of plastic to tame frizzy or flyaway hair, give body and bounce to fine hair or even make your hair defy gravity and stand straight up. They also reduce static electricity and keep hair cuticles tightly shut against moisture. This staves off the moment when humidity, mist, rain, perspiration or the next shampoo penetrates the cuticle, returning hair to its natural alpha state – frizziness for some people, lank limpness for others (see Chapter 5).

Unless you simply let your hair dry naturally, you need heat to fix your hair into the shape you desire – its beta keratin style, instead of its natural alpha keratin state. Use the right product for your kind of drying: **setting lotion** for rollers is too sticky for blow-drying. All the blow-dry products are fine for naturally drying your hair. **Blow-dry colour** gives a temporary hair colour, but its metallic ingredients may make treated hair turn orange or green; read instructions carefully!

Professional blow-drying secrets

1. Use a wide-toothed comb on clean, damp, conditioned hair to comb out tangles. Comb in styling product. Comb hair in direction of finished style.

2 Divide hair into workable major sections. Start at the nape and clip other sections out of the way.
3 For smooth, straight, medium or long styles, roll or pull hair on the styling brush, and aim drier nozzle at the roots first. This provides maximum volume and shape. Pull with even tension, but not too hard.
4 For casual, wild, full, layered or curly styles scrunch or finger dry using diffuser. Tip head forwards and dry hair from underneath to get lift at the roots. Grasp and ruffle sections of hair under the gentle heat.
5 Dry from roots towards ends to keep the cuticle closed flat, for best hair health and looks. Reposition brush carefully to avoid tangling.
6 Move the drier constantly, even as you concentrate on one spot, to prevent burning hair or scalp.
7 Dry each section thoroughly before moving to the next. Hot hair can feel damp, so give a cool blast before you decide whether it's dry. This helps close cuticles and hold the beta keratin style.

Professional roller-setting secrets

1 As 1 above.
2 Divide hair into sectors and clip out of the way. Make first roller section at the front of the head, keeping section lines very tidy, and the width a little narrower than the roller width.
3 Roll hair carefully on roller. Be sure ends are smooth and flat against the roller to avoid 'fishhook' ends when hair dries.
4 Roller should end up sitting directly on the roots, for best lift and bounce. Continue rollers towards crown, then work downwards.
5 Roll side and bottom rollers up for up-flicked hair, down for under-curves. Smaller rollers make hair curlier.
6 Let hair cool thoroughly before removing rollers.
7 Remove rollers from underneath first and work up, to avoid tangling. Handle unrolled hair gently.
8 Before final styling, brush hair thoroughly against direction of the set to remove roller marks.

Product lowdown: styling aids after drying

Finishing products give your hair healthy shine and lasting style.
Hairspray – spray no closer than 30 cm (1 foot) away to avoid build-up

– coats with a fine film of plastic to hold and shine. **Gel** (made of plant or seaweed gums plus plasticisers), **mousse** (oils and plasticisers) and **wax** (oils) hold, shine, control frizz and provide definition for curls or spikes, or they can slick, mould or sculpt hair with a wet or dry look. **Pomade** (of wax, oils) and **cream** (oils) provide a gentler hold than gels or waxes, and may condition hair. **Hair moisturiser**, **serum** or **activator** may be an oil spray or lotion which acts as a leave-in conditioner giving little hold, but great gloss, shine and static reduction. All of these products may contain vitamins, proteins and other rich conditioning ingredients, but their main function is to keep cuticles closed and add body and control.

> ### STYLE WOES: BEWARE OF BUILD-UP
> Styling products make 'good hair days' wondrously possible, but they cling and can eventually make your hair dull and heavy. Look for products which claim to brush out, and use a specialist clarifying shampoo now and then. See Chapter 5.

Perming and colouring

Thanks to chemicals – often thought of as a dirty word – you can have hair of just about any curliness or colour you desire. You can even, with care, change both curl *and* colour.

Ideally, you should have perms and colour done professionally in a salon. With specialist training, knowledge and products, a hairdresser provides more finished and predictable results than at home, and the process will be safer. But, of course, you can do it yourself – so long as you *always* follow the perm and colouring product instructions. These include directions for testing – do it!

Perm and colour success know-how

- **Virgin** is the hairdressers' term for hair that's never been chemically treated – no perms, no colour of any sort. It's the least risky hair to process.
- If you have coloured your hair and you want a perm, or visa versa, it's safest to go to a professional. If you must try both at home,

> ## SAFE AND HAPPY: USING CHEMICALS ON YOUR HAIR
>
> 1 Before you purchase perm or colour, perform the elasticity and porosity tests described on page 59.
>   If your hair fails either of these tests you should only have a professional perm or colour your hair.
> 2 Before you use perm or colour, 24 to 48 hours in advance, follow the pack instructions for testing a strand of your hair:
>   - for **incompatability** (will hair turn green, orange or break off?)
>   - for **curl** (how much curl will you get, after how long?) or
>   - for **colour** (what degree of colour will you get, after how long, will it take evenly?)
> 3 At the same time, 24 to 48 hours in advance, do the **skin patch** test, following instructions on the pack, for **sensitivity** (will your scalp burn or itch?)
> 4 Safety tips when you use perm or colour:
>   - Apply a barrier cream (like paraffin wax) around hairline to protect from chemical drips.
>   - Use plastic or rubber gloves supplied with kit.
>   - Cover up clothes and damageable surfaces.
>   - In case of accident, especially to eyes, flood the area with water. See GP, emergency clinic or, for less drastic situations, a hairdresser.

allow some time and good conditioning (see Chapter 5) between the two chemical assaults, read and follow manufacturers directions closely, and **do the tests**.

- Always be totally honest with your hairdresser about what you have put on your hair – some chemicals combine to create a disaster.
- Always use the special shampoos and conditioners that come with home perm and colour products. They are specifically made to work with the process.
- The front hairline is more porous than hair elsewhere; leave it until last when applying chemicals.
- The kindest cut. Get your hair cut or reshaped **after** perming or colouring, not before. For one thing, hair looks shorter after a perm, so you'll know what you're getting. For another, although it seems silly to cut off what you've just created, even the healthiest hair is porous at the ends and will show some damage; a trim's the best cure.

- Be extra gentle with hair for a week after applying a perm or strong hair-colour chemicals. They set out on purpose to damage your hair – that's how they do their work. Don't over-brush or use fierce blow-dry heat, tongs or hot rollers. To restore hair's health and shine after chemicals use extra-nourishing conditioners and perhaps a course of deep oil treatments or restructurants. See Chapter 5.
- Remember – you can restore your hair to a chemically untreated virgin state, if you have patience. Simply let it grow and cut off the chemically treated ends.

Product lowdown: permanent choices

So you've got kinks and long to have a curtain of straight hair? Or do you have stick-straight hair and long for rich waves? Hair's thin and limp, forever going flat? Or is it boringly well-behaved when you wish it were wild? Perms let you have hair that expresses your personal style.

Alkaline perms, with their ammonia smell and an acid balance of pH 9.5, are highly effective chemicals. (Remember, skin and hair are normally pH 5.4 to 6.2; see p. 62.) The newer **acid perms** (pH 5.5 to 7) are glyceryl based and need heat to help raise the cuticles; they're gentler and better for damaged hair.

Whichever kind you use, a perm permanently changes the strong alpha keratin bonds (the protein shape-controllers) in the hair cortex, and this lasts until the hair itself grows and the perm is cut off. Perms work by opening up the cuticles and softening the hair with a strong chemical lotion, then by moulding the hair to a new shape around the perm rods (curlers), and finally by fixing the new shape with a neutraliser.

Gone are the days when a perm automatically meant crimped or frizzy little curls. Spot perming and variations in rod size and placement allow a range of effects, for instance:

- Root perm – ends are left unpermed, by covering with cling film. Produces lift at roots to gives hair volume and bounce.
- Body wave – large rods give gentle waves and body, or hair can be blow-dried smooth. Good for layered short and medium or blunt-cut hair.
- Flex perm – smaller, flexible rods result in flowing waves or curls. Good on medium or long layered or straight-cut hair.

Straightening options

If you have naturally very tight, wiry curls (Afro-Caribbean or other), but you are looking for straighter hair, you can try one of the processes below.

Soft pressing – not permanent (the alpha keratin bonds in the cortex aren't changed), but the results of this heat-and-stretch styling process can last up to ten days. You need a hairdresser or friend to do it for you. Special oil or pomade protects hair and scalp from burning on the heated, metal pressing comb which slides through and stretches the hair small section by small section. Afterwards, hair is styled with curling tongs or blow drier. Soft pressing removes up to 70 per cent of curl; hard pressing, which simply repeats the process, can do more – but it can seriously damage hair.

Curly perm – a two-stage perm that starts with a curl rearranger which chemically straightens hair, then winds hair on perm rods and uses a milder chemical curl booster to create larger, softer curls. You can choose a wet or dry look.

Relaxing – a very strong perm (pH 10 to 14) that straightens hair which can then be set, blow-dried, etc. Hydroxide relaxers are the strongest, and remove curl. Thioglycollate (ammonium-based) straighteners reduce the degree of curl. Not only are these extremely harsh and risky to work with, but also the two kinds are a disaster together; you've got to grow out/cut off hair treated with one before using the other.

How permanent is a permanent?

When to re-perm? Once every six months, probably, but it depends on haircut and growth rates. Gentler acid perms may be renewed every four months, if desired.

What if the perm's a disaster? Go to a hairdresser. An uncurly perm can be re-permed with weaker solution, a too-curly perm can be gently relaxed, breakage or frizziness need a reconditioning course.

Product lowdown: colour choices

Platinum blonde, ravishing redhead, raven's wing, sunkissed – or simply hiding the grey? Whatever your personal style and hair-colour wish, be sure to take your own season colour group into account (see

Chapter 6). If you are a natural cool winter or summer you're unlikely to be flattered by a warm coppery hair colour. Likewise, a warm spring or autumn will find that ashen blonde hair does not do wonders for the face.

The degree of ageing on your face is a factor, too. A dark or ashy hair colour – even though you were born to it – can drain the complexion and age you further; go for softer shades. Beware: white hair will take on warm tones (red, copper) more brightly than other hair.

If you're feeling shy about breaking into colour, try a temporary colour first. Or try a colour very close to your own shade – it richly but subtly enhances your hair. Some colour treatment actually improves the texture, volume and behaviour of your hair, especially if it's thin, fine or lifeless.

When you're selecting a colour from the shelves or discussing it with your hairdresser, think about it in two dimensions. **Depth of colour** is how light or dark hair is: very light, light, medium, dark, very dark, black. **Tone of colour** is the shade of a given colour depth: ash, silver, golden, warm, red, copper. Put them together and you might have light warm brown or medium golden blonde or very dark copper ... the variety is endless. And then you have to think about how long you want the colour to last ... .

Temporary colour May be mousse, shampoo, rinse, setting lotion, hairspray. It goes on instantly, washes out with the next shampoo. The pigment simply coats the outside of the hair shaft; porous hair or a sprinkling of white strands will take colour, especially warm tones, strongly and wash out less easily. You can't lighten your natural hair colour with this, but you can darken, tone (ash/copper) or intensify your own colour. Ash blonde and silver shades are useful for lending a cleaner tone to grey or white hair that looks yellowish or dingy.

Semi-permanent Usually a shampoo, in the salon may be a mixed cream or a newer, low-strength, hydrogen peroxide formula. You apply it, wait until the colour develops, then rinse. Typically it lasts four to six shampoos and the colour fades gradually, so no margin of new root-growth shows. Some newer versions last through 12 shampoos, in which case roots may show. As above, porous hair will take the colour differently, and semi-permanent colour will not turn dark hair to blonde. It is best to use a shade near your natural hair colour. It's ideal for covering grey (but watch those red tones).

Permanent tints These colour your hair in one of three main won't-wash-out ways. One is natural – **henna** – but this is limited to copper and red tones. Another is **metallic dye**, sold as 'banish the grey' colour restorers; use thoughtfully, because if you perm, tint or bleach hair coloured this way, the hair will break off.

The most frequently used permanent colour, with the widest choice of colours, is **chemical dye** (**tint**) which is mixed with hydrogen peroxide – it may come as cream, gel or thick lotion. The alkaline formula tint opens the cuticle so the pigment enters the cortex; after the waiting period a special rinse closes the cuticle, and the dye is permanently trapped inside. Permanent tints allow you to go up to four shades lighter than your natural colour (see 'Permanent radical colour change', below, if you want to go even lighter). They also let you intensify or change your hair with a wide range of shades close to your own depth or darker. Chemical dyes are fine for grey hair, with the same red-shades warning.

Permanent radical colour change If you want a whole head of lighter hair or a colour too light for permanent tint, you have to bleach. This usually involves a mixture of oil or gel bleach, hydrogen peroxide and a sachet of powder that is the activator. The strong alkali raises the cuticles, the bleach lightens the natural colour pigments in the cortex. Hair lightens in this order: black, dark brown, red brown, golden brown, golden blonde, light blonde … hair will disintegrate if it gets beyond very light blonde. Rinsing stops the process at the shade of lightness you desire. If you wish, you then add your desired permanent tint (see above).

Highlights, streaks, lowlights These are permanent colour changes using bleach as for whole-head change, but with a subtle natural effect. One method used in salons or with home kits (you'll need a friend to help) is to pull strands (streaks) of hair through holes in a plastic cap. In salons, a more delicate effect comes from woven highlights, where alternate strands from locks of hair are picked up by a pin-tail comb and wrapped with foil strips as the bleach develops. Highlights and streaks are pale gold to flaxen. Lowlights are darker or more intensely toned (golden, copper, red, etc.) than the natural colour; this looks especially rich on dark blonde and brown hair.

The root of the problem

What about the colour as hair grows? Permanent tints, radical changes and highlights will show up your natural colour at the hair roots as hair grows. To keep your healthy good looks you need to retouch the roots with the tint or bleach – being careful not to overlap on to the previously treated hair. Otherwise hair will be damaged, possibly broken. If colour change is dramatic you may need to do this every four to six weeks. High/low lights are more subtle, so you can usually go for about four months.

What if you hate the colour? You can wash out temporary colour, and go mad with shampooing to fade semi-permanent colour. For a permanent tint, a colour stripper or reducer can save the day, but it's a professional job only. If bleached colour is too brassy or yellow you can try toning it down with a silvery or ashy temporary colour. Nothing can reverse bleach, but a professional can rebleach it or tint it.

What if the colour fades or changes? To prevent the bleaching effect of strong sun, use hair products with added sunscreens, especially in summer and on 'sun and sea' holidays. Sunscreens even protect natural hair colour.

— Hairstyle on a budget, in a hurry —

Money versus time

A *free* visit to the hairdresser? Yes, (or low cost) if you 'model' at a salon or hairdressing school, and you don't need model-girl looks. Watch for signs in windows or telephone to enquire. No spotlights and paparazzi, I'm afraid; they just want heads of hair for the stylist trainees to cut, style, colour, perm. You specify what you want, as you normally would, and it's done under a trainer's supervision by a student who already has some experience. You may gather useful information about your hair as the trainer reinforces the teaching. A few drawbacks: there may be only one time slot per week; some waiting around is inevitable while the trainer checks the work; next visit you'll probably get a different trainee.

Time versus money

If time is your main worry, consider a mobile hairdresser. She or he comes to your house, can even do the whole family. Look for local ads, ask friends or hairdressers if they can recommend someone.

HOW TO TRIM YOUR OWN FRINGE BETWEEN HAIR CUTS

Cling film sticks easily to your forehead, hangs down over your eyes to block off bits of hair, yet you can see what you're doing. Stretch sections of fringe vertically between fingers and snip slowly, checking results frequently. If you wet your fringe to make the hair hang straighter, remember that it 'shrinks' when it dries, so be careful how much you cut off!

Five hairstyling homebrews

Lemon-juice setting lotion Squeeze and strain juice, don't dilute, comb through hair.

Beer setting lotion Comb flat beer through hair before setting; adds body.

Camomile blonde-enhancer Steep two tablespoons of camomile tea in ½ litre (1 pint) boiling water and cool. Copiously rinse clean, wet hair with this after every shampoo. Over six to eight weeks blondeness is highlighted.

Sage or rosemary dark-hair enhancer Make and use in same manner as camomile rinse, above. Improves greying hair, too.

Home-made conditioning tips see Chapter 5.

BAD-HAIR-DAY RESCUES

- See 'Emergency Shampoo' tips, Chapter 5.
- Slap on mousse, gel or hairspray to restyle; maybe wear hair wet-look?
- Pull hair back with combs, hair slides or hairband.
- Put hair up in a casual bun or sleek pleat.
- Wear a hat, scarf or turban.
- Take the day off?

8

MAKING UP: FROM MINIMAL TO DRAMATIC

Here we are at the heart of beauty – or what most people think of as beauty – the colours and conjuring of make-up. Colour cosmetics, as the industry calls them, accentuate your looks and add flair to your style. Although you know that true beauty is health, make-up is the icing on the cake, the gilding on the lily, a lift to the spirits. How far do you want to go? It's a matter of personal style.

Five-stage self-assessment: what make-up style for you?

Make-up can take you from basic barefaced looks to making-a-statement drama. Whatever your personal style and varied lifestyle roles, you have the same make-up steps and products at your command. Step-by-step how-tos follow, but first, identify your make-up style of the moment. It's just a question of make-up by degree.

Minimalist: You're happy only to smooth your eyebrows, add a lick of eye definition (shadow *or* liner *or* mascara), a flick of blush and a dash of lipstick. Who needs the whole whack for playing tennis or minding the crêche? Or this basic four-degree look may be all you'll ever feel comfortable with if you're a born casual, natural, no-nonsense woman. (By the way, it can take ten make-up products to give a magazine model a 'natural' look.) NB: Actually, this is four-and-a-half degree make-up – be sure to start with a sunscreened moisturiser.

Subtle stylist: Minimal means a bit more to you. You're happy to add eyebrow pencil, mascara and some eyeshadow or liner, plus lipliner and lipstick. A lift of cheek colour, and that's six degrees of make-up (not counting moisturiser) to make you ready for work, a day in town, a bit of public interface. Still casual, but with an eye for flair.

Definitive stylist: You'll smooth on some light-textured foundation and maybe a dusting of powder, use two tones of eyeshadow plus liner, and all the six steps above to go up a notch. This is ten-degree make-up for town and business formality, maybe an evening out – or maybe you're only collecting the kids from school or seeing your doctor. Presentation does as much for your feelings about yourself as it does for your image in the actual situation. Make up, feel good!

Out to impress: You'll apply corrective underfoundation, three eyeshadow shades, liner, mascara, contouring, lip-shaping ... with this degree of make-up you're out to impress! Definitely for glam events; use subtle colours and careful blending, and you can even go this far for some work situations.

Dramatic: Brighter colours, heavy on the eyeliner, bold blush and shadow colours, gleaming highlighter, kohl eye pencil on the inner, lower eye rim, contrasting lipliner and lipstick. Superstar, punk, dramatic, fantasy ... day or night, this is Making A Statement.

Product lowdown: what make-up for whom?

There's a world of make-up to choose from. Category by category we'll cover choices in formulations, then choices in colours. After that, we'll look at the step-by-step in applying the make-up that's right for you.

Tooling-up for make-up

For good-looking make-up you need the right tools. Build up your collection gradually – long-handled brushes of natural hair give the best control, but they're pricey (however, they'll last a lifetime). Use pretty pots and little baskets to keep brushes, pencils, lipsticks, etc. to hand – and to make making up a mini-ritual and celebration of caring for yourself. Be hygienic, too; wash brushes, combs, sponges as needed.

Besides a mirror in good lighting, tissues, cotton wool, cotton swabs, hairband or clips you need:

- large, loose, soft brush for powder and blusher
- small, flat-shaped brush for eyeshadow
- smaller, stiff, short-cut brush for lipstick
- stiff, short brush/comb for eyebrows
- small, pointed brush if you paint on eyeliner
- pencil sharpeners for make-up pencils
- tweezers
- optional extras include eyelash curler, magnifying mirror, small natural sponges, spray spring water.

Make-up for skin

Foundation

The aim of foundation is to look like skin, so if you're happy with your bare skin, skip foundation. If you want to provide a smoother finish, even out skintones or cover freckles or blemishes, a foundation can help. Formulations with sunscreen provide vital protection from ageing, dangerous UV sunrays. Usually oil-and-water emulsions with pigments offer varied degrees of coverage.

Lightest coverage **Gel**, usually in a squeezy tube, gives thin, translucent colour, a warmth on bare skin.

Light to medium coverage **Liquid foundation**, in a bottle or tube, spreads easily (professionals call this playtime). **Mousse**, in an aerosol, is simply a very fine liquid which foams out to provide a sheer film of cover. Liquid foundations are good on *normal, combination and oily complexions*; you may wish to set richer formulae with powder. For *very oily or troubled complexions*, try **water-based liquid foundations** which contain extra absorbent ingredients; playtime is minimal, but foundations keep oily shine from breaking through. **Medicated foundations**, usually liquid, contain antibacterial ingredients to make them safer for use over spots or acne (ask your doctor, dermatologist or pharmacist to recommend a brand).

Medium coverage **Cream foundation**, in a jar or tube, has good playtime, plus humectants to provide extra moisture, so it's good for *dry skin*. You must usually set cream foundation with powder. Powder-cream compact blends like cream, but gives a powder finish.

Medium to heavy coverage **Cake foundation**, in a compact, is usually a compressed cream containing extra powder. It's most often applied with a damp sponge – wetter allows thinner coverage, drier heavier, ideal for *blemishes*. **Stick foundation**, often used by professionals, is firm enough to push up in a large lipstick-type tube; it gives ultimate coverage. Cake and stick foundation need powder afterwards.

Powder

Traditionally, you need powder only if you wear foundation. But you can wear it on bare skin: translucent shades reduce oily shine, tinted shades give sheer matt warmth. Water-based foundations can do without powder, but others benefit from an invisible dusting of it to set the oils in the formula, keeping your foundation base from melting or smearing.

Today's translucent powders are made of talc, and sometimes starch or silk. Professionals swear by loose powder applied with a brush – it's more hygienic and easier to control than pressed powder in a compact. If you don't usually wear full make-up you can get by with a compact powder – but use a big brush to pick up and apply the powder. Use the powder puff and compact for on-the-go touch-ups.

Conceal, correct, contour

Before, during or after you apply foundation (but before powder) you can use special products to help solve problems – but don't use these if they make you feel or look artificial. (Step-by-step guidelines follow later in this chapter.)

Concealer For *dark circles* and *blemishes*, concealer is a heavy-ish, foundation-type product which you buy in a shade lighter than your normal foundation. You could simply use a light foundation instead, although the covering power won't be the same.

Contourer Can give angles to a round face, soften an angular face, narrow a broad nose, create dramatic cheekbones. A brown contour product may be called a **shader or shaper**; soft white or frosted beige contourer is often called **highlighter**. Compressed powder, applied with a brush, is the easiest to use. Contourers also come as creams, or you can simply use foundations a notch lighter and darker than your basic shade – these methods are tricky to blend.

Correctors Underfoundations to improve complexion colour. If your *skin is very red*, or if you have blotchy areas of *fine veins*, use a **pale green**. If *sallow*, use **pinky-lilac**. You won't look like a clown; these lightly pigmented moisturising lotions or creams simply counterbalance skin tone under your normal foundation. If your skin is *very oily*, an **anti-shine formula** with absorbent ingredients helps to keep excess oil from breaking through your foundation. Usually you just need it on the 'oily T zone' of chin, nose and forehead.

Blusher

Blush gives a lift of freshness and colour to the face; you can also use it to contour. A **pigmented powder** pressed into a compact or into small balls or 'pearls', it's easy to apply with a brush on bare skin or after foundation and powder. **Bronzing powder** – loose or pressed – is midway between a blusher and all-over face colour. Blusher comes as **liquid**, **cream** and **gel**, too; you just have to experiment to see what you like. It's good to have two or three blush shades. (Colour suggestions follow later in this chapter.)

BEST BLUSH ALL-IN-ONE

Caught short on budget, time or space? Just one soft, brownish blush can work wonders. Use it on cheeks as usual, but also skim colour very lightly along the forehead hairline and on the tip of the chin. Brush it on to the outer eyelid and brow bone in place of eyeshadow. Tap the brush clean and go over the colour to blend well. *Voila:* a natural, co-ordinated, healthy-looking glow.

Make-up for eyes

Eyebrow pencil

If your brows are sparse or pale, a medium-soft eyebrow pencil matching your natural brow or hair colour lets you add the weight you need. Its 'lead' is made of a very stiff pigmented cream.

Eyeshadow

Colour-fun and shaping on the lids and browbones comes from eyeshadows as **creams**, **gels**, **pencils** and, most popular of all, **pressed powders**. Powders are the easiest to apply and blend; they're normally made with titanium dioxide for cover, oils for cling and spread, mineral or organic pigments for colour, and gum so they can be pressed into the metal pan (godet) in the compact. You might want a mini-wardrobe of colours, including lighter and darker shades for highlighting and contouring.

Eyeliner

A thin dark line just along the lashes accentuates the eye, although the look goes in and out of fashion. Some people do without eyeshadow and just wear liner. **Liquid liner** painted on with a thin, tapered brush needs a steady hand; it may come as a **cake** which you wet, as a sort of **felt-tip pen** or as a **liquid** with a gum ingredient for extra-dark shine. Pencil liner (sometimes call **kohl**) is smudgy to start with, so you can get away with wobbliness. Black, brown, grey, blue, green, purple, wine – you can be subtle or dramatic.

Mascara

Thick, dark lashes provide the ultimate basic eye appeal. Mascara once came only in a cake which you wet and applied with a little brush – many beauty and performance professionals still swear by this method. Far simpler is the automatic wand-brush in its own tube of mascara; the wand is the perfect tool and the mascara itself is made of pigments, resins, waxes, oils and water or water and alcohol. Some mascaras have protein conditioners, some have extra-thickening ingredients, some have fine fibres of nylon or rayon to add lash length (don't use this kind if you wear contact lenses). To avoid smudging and dark undereye circles, use waterproof mascara (and an oil-based mascara remover). Keep experimenting until you find a formula that works for you; mascara is among the most finicky of cosmetics to create, and one manufacturer's solution will be just right for you. Generally, stick to black or dark brown whatever your colouring; your aim is to emphasise – unless you want a dramatic touch of blue, green or violet.

False eyelashes

These are not for everyone, because they are fiddly to put on, feel strange to wear, look highly dramatic unless you're very skilful at application. But they are fun when you want to feel super glamorous or outrageous. Made of nylon or natural hair, they come in flexible strips which you trim to fit and attach with special adhesive to the base of your own lashes after applying all your other eye make-up. The trick is to squeeze some adhesive on to one knuckle, pick up the lash strip with tweezers and stroke the base lightly through the adhesive. With tweezers, position the strip very close to the natural lash base, centre first, then inner and outer corners. Let them dry for two minutes, then blend them with your own lashes using your eyebrow brush. Don't apply mascara afterwards as you can't clean them.

Make-up for lips

Lip pencil

This is lipstick with an extra amount of hard waxes to allow precise, long-lasting colour. Not everyone wants to bother, but you can use it to outline your natural lip shape to prevent lipstick bleeding into the skin near your lips, to reshape your lips, to make lip make-up last longer, or simply for a glamorous look. All you need is one or two shades very close to your lipstick colour and/or to your natural brown-red lip colour. For a dramatic look, try colour-contrasting lip pencil.

Lipstick

Contains pigments for colour, titanium dioxide for coverage, wax for firmness, oils for softness and spreadability. **Sheer** shades have less titanium dioxide than long-lasting **opaque** shades, **frosted** shades get their pearl from mica or other minerals. A lip brush gives you great-looking, long-lasting results and lets you use up every last bit of lipstick in the tube.

Lip gloss

This has lots of oils to give a shiny wet look to the lips. It may have no colour or some pigments and/or pearly ingredients. Use it over lipstick or on bare lips; unfortunately the melty, soft look doesn't linger long, so carry your wand or pot of gloss wherever you go.

THE BEST LIPLOOK SECRET

Lipliner in brownish, nearly natural lipcolour, and a slick of lipbrushed-on lipgloss – irresistably delicious and natural-looking lips.

Colours for your skin, eyes and lips

How to choose foundation and powder

1 Foundation names vary, but basically they're light, medium and dark, and within each depth you'll usually have choices of three main tonalities: warm (creamy, golden, honey, tan), neutral (ivory, beige, natural, olive) or heightener (rose, peach, bronze). Bear your season in mind. Cool winter and summer probably do well with neutral shades, or might try a tinge of livening pink. Warm spring and autumn should try warm shades first, though not stray too far into reddish tones. Brown and black complexions need dark beige, olive or bronze.
2 Before you test a foundation, check the skin on your inside arm, just above the wrist – is it the same colour as your complexion? If so, this is the spot to try on a foundation, *not* on the back of your hand which is bound to be darker and rougher than facial skin. If not, use your neck or your face itself to test colour.
3 Smooth on a streak of the shade you're trying, and look to see if it exactly matches the skin colour. It should practically disappear (except for the coverage it gives), showing no line where the colour starts. If you are pale-skinned you can possibly go one shade lighter than natural; if dark, possibly one shade darker. Remember, foundation is not meant to be a mask.
4 Always go to a window or outdoors to see the colour on your skin before making the decision. In-store lighting changes colours.
5 If foundation always turns orange on you, it means your skin is slightly less acid than average. Try a cooler, paler shade to allow for this difference.
6 Powder, used to set liquid, cream or cake foundation, should do its job invisibly, letting foundation colour show. Translucent, meaning one-neutral-shade-suits-all, is usually ideal. Some brands offer translucent light, medium or dark, subtly tinted to blend with foundation depth. The very darkest complexions should use only a brown, golden or bronze powder, to avoid a chalky look.

Make-up colours for your season and personal style

Generally your colour palette should tone with your season's skin and hair colouring (see Chapter 6), but within this there's room for a range of shades for your wardrobe, moods and occasions. Darker, brighter shades are dramatic; lighter, muted shades are subtle. For hot weather you might collect softer, warmer, translucent, frosted or glossy make-up.

Winters and summers

Winters, from silvery to bluey-brown in skin and hair tones, and summers, with their more delicate ash blonde, brown and grey hair and 'strawberries and cream' skin, need cooled, blue-toned colours.

- *Blush and lips* – pinks, roses, blue-reds, wines.
- *Eyes* – greys, blues, violets.

Summers need softened shades, such as dusty pink, smokey amethyst. Winters can wear more vibrant shades, such as hot pink, magenta, teal.

Autumns and springs

Autumns, with their ivory and golden beige skin, their chestnut-toned, red-blonde-brown or grey hair, and springs, with their fairer, golden honey or strawberry blonde colouring, need warm-toned colours.

- *Blush and lips* – corals, orange-reds, rusts and browns.
- *Eyes* – browns, tans, greens.

Autumns look good in earth colours such as olive green, terracotta. Springs shine in clearer shades such as camel, peach, pine.

Dark Asian, African, Afro-Caribbean and some Latina

These colourings provide opportunities for colourplay with deep and vibrant shades such as irridescent gold, bronze, copper, peacock and butterfly shades. They must still heed the basic warm (yellow-red) or cool (blue-purple) skin undertones, but for lip and cheek colours they can get away with really warm rich mango or pumpkin shades, or dazzling bright-cool fuchsia and plum. For less daring looks, browns, beiges and burgundies are their classics.

Trendy and classic

Whatever your colouring and season, if you're a trendy beauty you'll add new fashion shades as they suit you or outrageous shades just for fun. If you want minimal fuss, whatever degree of make-up you wear, you need only stock up – always sticking to the cool or warm tonality that flatters you – on colour cosmetics' all-purpose *classics*:

- red lipstick
- soft brown blush
- eyeshadows/liner in browns-tans for autumns and springs, or in greys for winters and summers
- dark brown mascara.

Make-up ages and stages

As years creep on, tone make-up down: hair colour and even skin colour may fade from the late forties onwards; check to be sure your foundation and make-up colours still suit you.

- Don't get stuck in a time warp, wearing the same eye and lip colour when you're 58 that you wore when you were 28. Review current make-up looks and adapt to your personal style.
- Use lighter-textured foundation and a minimum of powder to avoid clogging in wrinkles and crevices.
- It's best to forgo contouring and bright eye and cheek colours, although you may need to thicken and darken eyebrows and lashes.
- Don't use frosts and glosses; they highlight wrinkles.
- Play around with lip colours – too dark and they look hard, too light and you look washed out. Lip pencil is a must, to keep colour from bleeding into tiny wrinkles around the lips.

Coping with scars and birthmarks

It's not easy to live with these. Through a dermatologist, hospital clinic, beauty salon or self-help organisation (see the list at the end of this book) you can get advice on special extra-covering foundations which blend perfectly with your skin colour, and lessons in how to use them. Do be sure to draw attention to your assets and cultivate your personal style (Chapter 6).

Your personal make-up style

First, shape your eyebrows

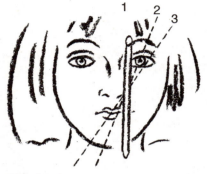

Figure 9 Find your ideal eyebrow

Brows give emphasis and expression to the face, and they frame the eyes. Thick, heavy brows can be very handsome – or they can glower and reduce the eye area. Thin, high brows may give a delicate look – or a bare look of constant surprise. Yours may be just right, although make-up and eye definition always benefit from a tidying.

Plucking hairs from the eyebrows may hurt a bit, and it may leave the area pink and tender for a while. But you have to do it this thoroughly only once, and ever afterwards you just need to remove the odd newly sprouted hair.

What shape should you aim for? Your own face tells you.

1 Align a long-handled brush or a pencil vertically along the side of your nose. Where it crosses the eyebrow is where the eyebrow should start. Remove hairs growing towards the bridge of the nose for wide, well-defined eyes.
2 Slant the pencil from the side of your nose on a line across your iris to cross your eyebrow – this is the highest point of the brow. You may want to shape an arch by removing hair from beneath the eyebrow. Never pluck from above it: you want to open up eye space, not bear down on it.

3 Slant the pencil even further, so it crosses the outer corner of your eye on its way to the eyebrow. This reveals its ideal end. Remove hairs beyond this point to avoid the look of droopy eyes.

Gradually remove one hair at a time, pausing often to brush and check the effect. Switch back and forth between both brows, to be sure to keep them even. You might want simply to tidy up, or to style thicker or thinner eyebrows, straighter or arched, tapered or not – study magazine pictures and people around you to help you decide. Generally, very thin brows and very angled ones look unflatteringly harsh, so go easy. When you've finished, go over the entire browbone area to remove the very fine nearly invisible hairs – this gives a remarkable yet subtle definition to the eye area, and allows make-up to go on more easily.

Plucking tips

- Make tweezing kinder by warming the eyebrow area with a hot face flannel. Heat relaxes the follicle area so it lets go of the hair more easily.
- Afterwards, soothe the area with alcohol-based toner or witch hazel; possibly rub with an ice cube to close pores. Don't use eye make-up until pinkness fades.
- Take out the minimum to achieve tidiness and shape; the hair follicles in this thin-skinned region are delicate and hair may not regrow, leaving you with permanently thin brows. (If this is already the case with you, consider micropigmentation, see Chapter 11.)
- Don't ever shave eyebrows – they grow back stubbly, straggly and stronger than ever. Don't use depilating cream either; it's far too dangerous near the eyes.

Your step-by-step make-up plan

Bare minimum? Business presentation? Dining out? Best tiara? Whatever the occasion the steps are the same, it's just a question of degree and colour choice. Minimalists and Subtle Stylists will start with Step 6 below and pick and choose among 7, 8 and 9 before finishing with 10 and 11. Definitive Stylists and *N*th-Degree make-up believers are likely to take all 12 steps.

THREE FOOLPROOF MAKE-UP TIPS

- **Automatic blender** You want no harsh lines of colour, just subtle shading. That's why brushes are so brilliant. After applying colour, wipe the brush with a tissue and use the clean brush to blend make-up to a whisper.
- **Smeary deary**... After you load up your shadow or blush brush, tap off excess before applying the colour. Place a tissue under your eye on your cheekbone to prevent dustings of eyeshadow or blodges of mascara from messing up your make-up. Use a cotton swab and a tiny bit of moisturiser to dab up smears.
- **Stay sharp** Ideally, sharpen your eye, lip, etc. pencils before each use; a slightly rounded point works well, though brow pencil should be fine or chisel-pointed.

Step 1 Foundation

Clip or pull hair off face. Face should be freshly cleansed and moisturised. If you choose a complexion corrector, dot the cream or lotion over skin and use your fingertips to blend in.

Use foundation directly from the bottle, tube or compact, or pour a little into one hand. Use fingertips or a small dry-damp sponge (squeeze out water, then blot it in tissues), dab a few splodges of foundation on your forehead, blend over skin, up to hairline and out to temples, with fingers or sponge. Dab a bit more on one cheek and spread under eye and downward; repeat on other side. Continue with sides of nose, up over nose and onto eyelids and bone. Then work around lip area, chin and jawline. Smooth some foundation under the jaw to feather out the colour.

Don't massage foundation into skin, just lightly pat, dab, smooth. Unlike skincare application, where you always move upwards, apply foundation in downward and outward strokes, going with, not against, the growth of fine, downy hairs on the face.

Step 2 Concealer

If you want to diminish dark circles, spots, crow's feet, brow furrows, deep smile lines, now pat on concealer – either a lighter shade of foundation or a cream or stick a shade lighter than your foundation. Don't drag a stick over the skin, instead dot on and gently pat with fingers.

If you want to shape and contour with cream shader and highlighter, do it now (see Steps 5 and 10).

Step 3   Powder

To set the foundation, use your biggest lushest brush to dust loose powder all over your face. Go lightly, don't scrub it in. Tap and wipe powder off the brush and go over the face again to remove all excess powder. If you don't invest in loose powder, brush over the surface of pressed powder to dust on a nearly-as-good matt finish that makes foundation last.

Step 4   Naturalising the look

Now settle it all and remove any obvious excess. Dampen a tissue with a spray of water and lay it on your face. Press it gently over every area. Blot, don't rub. You could instead spray your face directly with a fine aerosol of spring water and lay a tissue over this, or you could blot with a dry-damp sponge. As well as naturalising the look and feel, this step helps foundation last longer.

Step 5   Contouring

Optional face contouring with powder shader and highlighter is only for those who wear full make-up, and even then probably only for evening and artificial lighting. You must blend skilfully and subtly, or you'll look like you've got stripes on your face. To blend, you must use cream contourers *before* applying face powder, or powder contourers *after* face powder. The visual law of design is your guide: dark diminishes, light lifts.

Slim a broad nose: Shade down sides of nose, light down the centre.

Shorten a long nose: A touch of dark at the tip.

Contour a round or square face: Shader at sides of forehead and at jaws. Add highlighter: down centre for round face to add length; on centre chin only to soften square face.

Enhance a small or large face: Outside the cheeks and temple add highlighter to enlarge, or shader to cut down size effect.

Dramatic interest: Shade hollows in cheeks from just under the upper jawbone slanting down on to cheeks, highlight cheekbones.

Step 6 Eyebrows

Brows frame and contain eyes, and eye make-up mustn't overwhelm them. See eyebrow-shaping section on page 118. Brush your brows with an eyebrow brush to remove any foundation and powder and to smooth the hairs. If you have dark brows this may be all you need – if they're unruly slick on a little petroleum jelly or clear mascara. For thin or pale brows sketch colour on to existing hairs and draw tiny hair-like strokes to thicken or extend the brows. Don't draw a hard continuous line – it looks artificial. Try using two eyebrow pencil shades (red-brown with brown for redheads, light-brown with grey for blondes, etc.) for the most realistic effect.

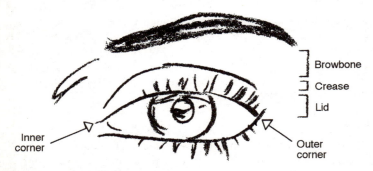

Figure 10 Eyeshadow application

Step 7 Eyeshadow

Choose two or three toning eyeshadow shades – pressed powder shadows to apply with a brush, or pencils to smudge with your fingers or a smudger. Cover the eyelid first using a medium shade, working from the inner corner towards the outer. Apply shadow to your eyes in parallel, one shade at a time. Work upwards, generally putting darker shadow just above the crease of the socket, blending it smoothly into the lid colour. Blend a lighter colour or shadow highlighter on the browbone, melding it into the darker crease shadow. Here are some tricks for particular kinds of eyes:

Prominent eyes: Muted shadow all the way from lashes to browbone, tiny bit of highlighter on browbone. No frosted shades; soft liner and lots of mascara.

MAKING UP: FROM MINIMAL TO DRAMATIC

Deep set eyes: Lightish shadow on lid blending to lighter on browbone. No dark at creases. Highlighter or light shade on centre of lids. Keep eyebrows tidy, not heavy.

Small eyes: Light on lid, dark on socket line, light on brow and highlight in centre of lid. Just beneath the eye apply a small smudge of dark colour from outer corner to centre, leaving about 1 mm uncovered below the lower rim.

Close- or wide-set eyes: To open space between eyes use a light shade at the inner corner and blend in darker shadow from centre of lid outwards and upwards. To narrow the space if the bridge of your nose seems too broad, do the opposite: dark at inner corners, light from centre outwards.

Hooded eyes: Darkish shadow at inner corners, blended to above outer corners (not following lash base). Highlight browbone and use the small-eyes undereye smudge trick.

Step 8   Eyeliner

Eyeliner is optional with eyeshadow. It can also stand alone. Use it for subtle, natural, eye emphasis or sophisticated effects. Start at the inner corner of the eyelid and draw the line close to the lash base. You can also draw a line on the lower lid below the lashes. Liquids paint on a hard line for dramatic looks. Pencils give a smudgier effect. The line can begin halfway along the eye, be extended beyond the outer corner, or be a series of stippled dots ... experiment!

Step 9   Mascara

An eyelash curler looks like an instrument of torture, but it'll flick up your lashes for better eye emphasis – use it alone or before mascara.

To mascara upper lashes, hold mascara wand horizontally. If you gently 'blink' your lashes through the wand brush you can get good coverage on both sides of the lashes. Otherwise, half-close your eye and stroke mascara on upper side of top lashes, then open wider and stroke colour on the underside. Do one coat and separate lashes with an old dry wand or eyebrow comb/brush; add second coat when dry – this builds up thickness without clumping.

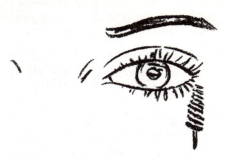

Figure 11 Use mascara wand vertically for lower lashes.

Don't forget lower lashes! Hold wand vertically and paint mascara on to these tiny but eye-defining lashes. Remember to cover outer corner lashes, too.

Step 10 Blusher

Blusher has been left until now, so you can see how much (or little) to use with your eye make-up – eyes should dominate. Usually you want a gentle glow of fresh radiance; always blend so the blush doesn't show as patches or lines. Powder blush is the easiest to manage, whether on bare skin or after foundation and powder. Use creams or gels only on bare skin or on foundation before powder (apply and blend with fingertips).

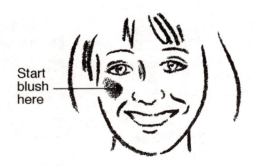

Figure 12 Blusher: smile and find the apple of your cheek.

Smile brightly, and you'll see the 'apple', the highest point of the cheek, below the middle of the eye; drop your smile and lightly start your blush stroke here, crescenting the colour upwards, fading it on to the temple. You might want to use a darker, brown-toned blusher in the hollows of your cheeks for more definition (see Step 5, Contouring).

Step 11   Lips

Lips are the main focus of the face, after eyes. Lipcolour looks and lasts best if you start with lip pencil. Simply draw from centre to corners of top lip, then bottom lip. Then fill in the lips with lipstick or gloss – but for really great looks, use a lip brush to paint on lipstick and to blend in the lipliner. If all this is too much trouble for you, a simple dash of lipstick straight from the tube is one of the world's quickest and easiest ways to flaunt some style.

For the longest-lasting colour, after application use a clean tissue to dust some face powder over the lipstick (before gloss), then blot lips on a tissue. Then apply lipstick again and/or gloss. Some lip cheats:

Thin lips: Widen with lipliner slightly outside the natural lip line. Use bright or glossy lipsticks.

Thick lips: Narrow with lipliner just inside the natural lip line. Avoid gloss and frosts.

Uneven lips: If size or natural colour are unbalanced use slightly lighter and darker tones of the same lipstick shade (light to lighten and enlarge, dark to deepen and downplay).

All of the above: Try applying foundation over lips before any lip make-up, then do the lip correcting – you would probably only do this for evenings and high drama.

Step 12   Finishing touches

Do your hair, put on your earrings, spray on your fragrance – you're gorgeous!

Face accessories – accents for your face and make-up

Earrings – coloured, dangly, tailored, classic pearls, natural shells, heirloom, made-it-yourself? Ear lobes only, or multi-pierced? Use earrings to co-ordinate your look, to accentuate your personal style.

Nose stud – not everyone goes for this, but lots do, another chance to attract interest and to make a statement.

Hair ornaments – hairbands, combs, hair slides, pony-tail ties, turbans, scarves all accentuate the face and total look; choose according to your season and personal style.

Eyeglasses – generally, choose frames that are opposite to your face shape (round or oval frames for angular faces, angular frames for rounded faces). Fashions in frames come and go, so you may want larger or smaller, coloured plastic or metal frames – take your time when choosing and keep your wardrobe and season in mind: silver and cool colours for winters and summers, gold and warm colours for autumns and springs. Glasses draw attention to the eyes, a plus for eye make-up.

Contact lenses – all eyeglass wearers should give contact lenses a try; manufacturers are making them easier and easier to wear. They come in colours, too, so you can intensify your washed-out blues or cloudy hazels, or perhaps change eye colour completely.

Sunglasses – although they cover the eyes they're a sophisticated accessory for practicality or for fun.

On-the-go beauty

Leave the house at 7:30 a.m. and don't get back until 10 p.m? Carry a small make-up bag containing:

- hairbrush (or hair pick/Afro comb for curly-heads)
- powder blush
- pressed powder compact if you wear foundation
- lipliner
- lipstick (gloss)
- tissues to blot oily shine.

Day-into-night beauty for that after-6 event

To the above list add:

- mousse, gel or hairspray; maybe hair slides, combs or elastic.
- mascara, eye-liner, brighter eyeshadows – make the eye-make-up more intense, thicken those lashes
- brighter, glossier lipstick – apply with lip brush
- a change of earrings, necklace, brooch or scarf
- a change of fragrance: richer, bolder.

GIVE YOURSELF A QUICK NEW LOOK

Bend over and brush hair so it's full and bouncy, or scoop it up to show profile and nape, or wet-look it slick or sculpted.

Bridal, portrait and television make-up

Here comes the bride

If you are planning a full, white wedding (even if your dress is pink or gold or ...) make your skincare, hair, make-up part of the plans.

- Consider your season when you try on dresses; pure white suits cool winter and summer skin tones, warmer cream is better for autumn and spring colouring.
- Try various hairstyles with your chosen headdress and veil – up, down, curled, smooth? It should be special but still you, and it's got to last through a long, exciting day. If you are going to have your hairdresser do your hair for the big day, take along the headdress and have a trial run, or at least a discussion.
- Get your skin into glowing, radiant condition. Plan a series of treatments in the six weeks leading up to the wedding. But do not use masks and deep cleansing treatments during wedding week because impurities may rise to the surface on the day itself. Tweeze eyebrows in advance, too.
- Have a make-up trial run. This is probably the only time in your life you'll wear a veil or be extensively photographed: what colour lipstick, how much eyeshadow? The day itself is no time to experiment.

- To help make-up last on the wedding day use translucent powder to keep shine controlled, blot with a dry-damp tissue, use the lasting lipstick routine described in the step by step.
- Having a formal bridal portrait done in advance gives you a chance to try out the whole look. See 'Watch the birdie' below.
- Schedule a course of manicures to shape up hands – they're centre stage as you hold the flowers, remove the veil, show off the ring, cut the cake.

Watch the birdie

Whether it's a passport photograph or a formal portrait, camera lighting can do harsh things – wash out assets, create lines and circles. To avoid disaster, use a light foundation to even out skin tones and create an unshiny matt surface. Prevent shadows with meticulously blended paler foundation or concealer under eyes, on smile creases and chin crease. Contour structure in the face with shader in hollows of cheeks. Strengthen eye definers; avoid the glare of pearlised eyeshadow colours. Lipcolour should be medium to light – bright and dark shades look harsh. Don't let a fringe overshadow your face; sweep it back, to one side, curl it or trim it.

If you're over 35 and have a say in things, ask for flat lighting and over-exposure to fade wrinkles out of existence. All this make-up feels, and in daylight looks, mask-like and trollopy, but in that frozen photographic image it works.

Fifteen minutes of fame

Super-bright television studio lighting is a challenge. Make-up and hair problems and solutions are the same as for still photography, although your movement, smiles, talk will help by animating your face.

Clothes are important. Wear solid red or another strong, bright colour in your season (such as yellow, turquoise, pink) even if it's not your usual style, because pale colours bleach you out, dark colours turn to black, checks and busy patterns dazzle the camera. Wear a two-piece outfit so microphone wire can go on easily. Choose a neat, unfussy design that fits well, doesn't bunch up or wrinkle when you sit; check your profile look as the camera will see you. Go for an uncomplicated neckline for those camera close-ups, and lighter-weight fabric because of the heat under the lights. You'll be a star!

What a professional can do

At a clinic or salon you'll get:

- Intensive, knowledgeable skincare (detailed in Chapter 4); good skin is essential before make-up.
- Eyelash and eyebrow tinting. Ideal if eye make-up is difficult for you (allergies, contact lenses, can't bear the fuss), or if you're a sportswoman or off to a hot climate. The dye uses peroxide and is permanent until hairs grow out in six to eight weeks. This should not be done at home, **never** done with normal hair dyes; it's close to your eyes – a job only for professionals. Note that eyelash tint does not thicken or curl lashes, so if you like a made-up look, you still need mascara.
- Eyebrow shaping – thoroughly. If you're unsure about what shape or how to do it, you could get your first shaping, or a new one, done at a salon. They often use rapid-action automatic tweezers, and you will be able to lie back in comfort while the job is done.
- Removing or bleaching facial hair, removal of fine veins, see Chapter 9.
- Make-up 'before and after' lessons, advice on products, make-up for weddings and special events. You can even book a make-up artist to come to you.

MAKE-UP RESCUE

You can deal with bad hair days – what about bad face days? Some quick fixes for droopy, drained, disastrous looks caused by colds, hayfever, late night partying, baby-broken nights, stress or heartbreak:

- Start the day with exfoliating facial scrub to wake up glow-giving microcirculation.
- Try an instant 'beauty lift' product: firms, tautens, brightens skin.
- Use concealer cream on bags and circles.
- Distract attention away from undereye circles by using deeper colour on eyelids, no mascara or liner beneath the eye.
- Use blusher generously.
- Gloss lips for softness and moist shine.
- Wear your best colour, or a bright scarf or interesting brooch.
- If it's the only way out, wear sunglasses!

9

TOP TO TOE: TOTAL BODYCARE

'Hands, fingers, knees-and-toes, knees-and-toes' – the children's song spotlights lots of good-looks assets, beyond face and hair. This is the category the beauty industry calls top-to-toe, and there are plenty of stops along the way.

The nose knows: the art of fragrance

Product lowdown: perfume and friends

Perfume enhances your feel-good factor and projects your personal style. A fine perfume may have more than 200 ingredients, the blend created by a 'nose', a highly trained and sense-gifted expert. The fragrance is always developed as a perfume, from which springs the product variants: eau de toilette, soap, body spray, body lotion, etc. Properly speaking, only perfume itself can be called **perfume**; it lasts the longest because it has the most essential oils, which make it the most expensive form to produce and to buy. Generally, **eau de toilette** (edt) spray is the easiest to wear and apply; it lasts up to four hours.

There's an art to choosing a fragrance for yourself. You must go further than the initial appeal to find fragrances that suit your body chemistry, for you have your own 'invisible' scent as individual as a fingerprint. A combination of the acid/alkaline balance of your skin, of body oils, perspiration, hormones, diet and lifestyle factors, your body chemistry subtly affects a fragrance, so what smells great in the magazine sample or on your best friend may not work for you. Body chemistry can also lift and project a fragrance, making it uniquely yours.

Your personal style in fragrance

Collect a small wardrobe of favourites: for day, evening, summer; for moods dreamy or upbeat.

Class	Description	Examples
Green	The lift of new-mown grass, sap, leaves. Tangy, vibrant.	Vent Vert (Balmain), Y (St Laurent)
Single floral	The impression of one flower, say lily of the valley, tuberose, or rose. Innocent, fresh.	Muguet des Bois (Coty), Diorissimo (Dior)
Floral bouquet	Blend of flowers, like rose and jasmine or gardenia and violet. Luxurious, sophisticated.	Joy (Patou), Chloe (Lagerfeld)
Fruity	Combination of orange, lemon, perhaps peach, melon. Rich, indulgent.	Anais, Anais (Cacherel), Giorgio (Giorgio)
Chypre (means cypress, pronounced *shee-pra*)	Medley of smoky oakmoss, amber, sandalwood. Distinctive, warm.	Ma Griffe (Carven), Femme (Rochas)
Oriental	Heady blend of musks and florals. Sensuous, intense.	Shalimar (Guerlain), Opium (St Laurent)
Modern (technical name: aldehyde)	Complex floral spicy impression, unidentifiable because of the chemist-perfumer's craft. Sparkling, romantic.	Chanel No 5 (Chanel), Arpège (Lanvin)

Six steps to finding your own signature fragrance

Buy only the real thing, only from bonafide outlets. Cheap fragrances and street-vendor fakes turn into weird and nasty smells. Assess fragrances the way industry professionals do to discover what works best on you.

Step 1 Don't decide by a sniff right from the bottle; you'll mostly get a whiff of alcohol, the dilutant.

Step 2 Spray or dab fragrance on your wrist, or the back of your hand or arm, or inner elbow. Wave your hand about for a moment to let the alcohol evaporate. Now begins the dry-down.

Step 3 Try one fragrance at a time, at most four in widely spaced places on your skin. The sense of smell is finely tuned and can get tired or confused.

Step 4 Don't judge immediately. The first bloom of scent on the skin is the top note. It's all-important for the sheer pleasure of putting on the fragrance, but it won't last long.

Step 5 Check the smell of the fragrance(s) on your skin after half an hour, then an hour. This is the longer-lasting middle note, which lingers into the day or evening.

Step 6 Much, much later, see what's left of the fragrance. It may be a hint of muskiness or a tinge of woodiness. This is the base-note, the foundation which sustained the fragrance. It may even cling until morning.

— A beautiful gesture: handcare —

Do you want your nails short and practical? Long and colourful? Do you have nails to speak of? Your hands can be a good-looks asset, or they can detract from your overall impression. Even if yours aren't elegant they can still be well groomed.

Hand and nail know-how

Healthy handcare starts by protecting your hands from everyday exposure to water, soap, detergents, cold, heat, daylight, and the grime and battering of house cleaning, gardening, job, sports or hobbies. Wear rubber gloves for the dirty work, warm gloves in winter, and keep a tube or bottle of hand-cream here, there and everywhere (kitchen, bathroom, bedside table, desk drawer, car, handbag) so you can massage in replenishing moisture and lubrication any time. The skin of the backs of your hands has a structure like the skin of your face, and hands show age as much as or more than your face, so use sunscreened lotion on them. An easy way to do this is simply to use your face moisturiser on your hands.

To maintain good-looking fingernails, it helps to know what they're made of. Like hair, fingernails are dead and made of keratin. The living part, the **matrix**, is the source of nail cells; the half-moon (**lunula**) on your thumbnails is a glimpse of it. Normally, natural oils and moisture keep nails flexible and firm; frequent use of water and detergents depletes the oils and leaches the moisture, causing dry, brittle, flaking or splitting nails. The **cuticle** is a small, thin extension of skin that clings protectively to the base of the growing nail. It should be soft and pliable, but it, too, can get dry and hard, and may split to become a hangnail.

Finally, nails say a lot about your overall health. They're the last stop on a sort of conveyor belt of nutrition and circulation: poor eating, stress and illness show up as weak, thin nails or as horizontal nail ridges. On a day-to-day basis, you can help nails and cuticles by rubbing your hand-cream into them, and by pushing back your cuticles as you do so.

Nail facts

- Fingernails grow on average 1 mm ($^1/_{32}$ in) per week. Toenails grow more slowly.
- To help weak, flaking nails, try a one-to three-month course of gelatine capsules and/or vitamins and minerals including extra B, A and E.
- White spots on the nail are usually due to minor injury; they grow out harmlessly. Their presence on every nail may mean a calcium or zinc deficiency.
- Buffing helps nails grow faster because it stimulates circulation. So does typing and piano-playing.
- Nail-biters who chew nails, cuticles and skin around nails risk finger infection. Break the habit with manicures, bitter-tasting nail paint, gradual reduction to gnawing only one finger.

Product lowdown and tooling-up: nail care

Raving red talons or short 'n' simple, a modest stock of items will help keep nails snag-free and attractive.

- **Emery boards** Never use metal ones; they're too harsh.
- **Orange sticks** Made of orange wood which is soft yet unsplintery. Pointed end is for cleaning, bevelled for pushing back cuticle. You can also buy a rubber-tipped hoof stick for pushing.
- **Cuticle cream** An emollient for softening and lubricating cuticles, making them pliable enough to push back easily.
- **Cuticle remover** An alkaline liquid with moisturiser to break down old cuticle clinging to the nail plate. It can bleach nails, too. It is strong, so follow instructions and rinse well.

Also: **nail scissors** or **clippers**, **cotton wool**, **warm water**, **soft nail brush**, **hand** or **body lotion**.

For non-enamel manicure

- **Nail white pencil** Contains titanium dioxide to whiten underside of nail's free edge.
- **Nail buffer** A pad covered with chamois leather.
- **Buffing paste** Optional cream which contains an abrasive (such as silica or chalk) to give natural sheen and smooth out nail ridges.

For nail-enamel manicure

- **Oily nail enamel remover** Acetone is the usual solvent, but it's extremely drying. Buy remover containing oils or glycerol, or an acetone-free formula.
- **Nail mender** Optional, for perfectionists only. See Step 5a, in 'Your step-by-step manicure plan', below.
- **Coloured polishes** These are made of film-forming plastics, oils to give flexibility, pigments for colour, formaldehyde to give gloss and solvents which evaporate to let the enamel dry. Old nail polish goes thick and takes longer to dry; hot and damp weather slow drying, too. Pale colours may need only one coat, pearly colours need no top coat, and some brands say they're one-coat only.
- **Base coat** Has ingredients similar to polish, but without pigment, to paint on first to provide a smooth surface and to prevent staining nails. May be a ridge-filler formula.

- **Top coat** As base coat, but more sealing power to protect coloured enamel from chipping.
- **Quick-dry spray** Optional aerosol solvent with conditioners to speed enamel drying rate. Natural drying is superior.

Your step-by-step manicure plan

If you wear nail enamel (some call it varnish or lacquer; it's said Charles Revson, founder of Revlon, would fire anyone who called it polish), you need a manicure once a week. If you wear bare nails, Steps 2 to 5 every other week will keep your nails healthy and good-looking. You can't rush a full nail-enamel manicure – allow an hour for Steps 1 to 8, maybe watch TV or listen to music during drying time.

Step 1

Assemble all your equipment. Remove old enamel by soaking a piece of cotton wool in remover and pressing it on each nail, holding it down for two to three seconds. This softens the enamel. Then go over each nail, wiping colour away; repeat. Rinse hands.

Step 2

Shape nails with the rough side of an emery board. If you want to shorten nails, use clippers or scissors first, then the emery board. Even if your nails are exactly right, file them to remove the thin, worn ends and to keep nails strong. **Always** work from one side of a nail toward the centre, in one direction only; back-and-forth filing weakens the nail. Don't file low down at the sides, for the same reason.

What shape? Short, square nails are practical, longer squared nails (with rounded corners to prevent breakage) enhance tapering fingers, an oval shape is generally attractive. Pointed nails look vampirish and break off easily. Finish off your shaping with the smooth side of the emery board.

Step 3

Apply cuticle cream to the base of each nail, massaging it in. Soak both hands in a bowl of warm water for a few minutes. Wrap a bit of cotton wool around the bevelled end of the orange stick, dip it in warm water, and gently push the cuticles back. If cuticle clings to the nail, apply cuticle remover with the cotton-wrapped point of the orange stick, and use the bevelled end to push cuticle away. Rinse off remover; push back cuticles again. The goal is neat, clear nail edges (if cuticles or hangnails are difficult, have a professional use cuticle clippers – a job for an expert only).

Step 4

Apply hand-cream and work it well into your hands.

Step 5

For non-enamel wearers – if you're happy with plain nails, dampen a nail-whitening pencil with water and run it under the free edges of nails. Then buff nails with or without a tiny dab of paste polish. Buff briskly but lightly in one direction only, from base to free edge, about 20 strokes per nail.

Step 5a

For nail-enamel wearers – dampen cotton wool with nail enamel remover and wipe down each nail to remove creams and help polish adhere. If you pride yourself in your perfect manicure, mend any split nails with an instant acrylic nail strengthener or hardener, or a patching kit of fibrous tissue and special adhesive, following manufacturers' instructions. Cover the mend in the next step.

Step 5b, 6, 7, 8

Apply base coat, two coats of nail enamel, and a coat of top coat, one thin layer at a time. The method is the same for each: only three quick strokes for each nail – centre, side, side – from base to tip. Wait until each coat is thoroughly dry (touch to see) before applying the next. Otherwise the finish dents or smudges.

Lasting power

A good nail-enamel manicure will last for about three days before edges wear and a little growth shows at the base. Slick on another coat of coloured enamel; two to three days later slick on another. After this, or if enamel chips, remove all enamel and start again.

Great looks for nails: your choices

- What colour nail enamel? 'Matching lips and fingertips', introduced in the 1940s by Revlon, is great fun and a brilliant marketing ploy to double-up cosmetic purchases. Ploy or no, it is a good idea to keep your nail shade in the same family with your lipcolour. Another route is to choose a classic go-with-all light pink or coral, or standard sexy red (within your cool or warm season).

- If you want to play down hand or nail problems don't use bright, dark or frosted shades.
- A **French manicure** gives a look between natural and full elegant enamel: use white pencil or enamel on the free edge and a very pale tinted translucent nail enamel over the entire nail.
- **False stick-on nails** can be fun for special events, or to rescue one single broken nail in your own otherwise perfect set. They need to be shaped, filed after gluing on to nails, then enamelled. Follow manufacturers' instructions.
- If you're seriously into gorgeous nails, see a specialist professional for **gel**, **tips**, **sculptured nail extensions**, **nail wraps** ... they take up to an hour to apply and need monthly salon revisits but they're remarkably permanent. Some can be worn without nail enamel, or you can go 100 per cent the other way and decorate them with dramatic patterns.
- **Allergies?** Some people react to nail enamels (usually it's the formaldehyde). Itching, swelling, redness, blisters, and dry, flaky skin show up not at fingertips, but at places you touch frequently, often the eye area, mouth, neck, chest. Give up polish or look for a non-formaldehyde formula.

On your toes: footcare

Foot and toenail know-how

Summer's the time when your feet are on show, but they need maintenance all year round. To prevent problems:

- A daily bath, shower or foot-wash helps prevent smelly feet and infections. If your feet perspire a lot, try frequent hosiery changes, special foot antiperspirants, deodorised insoles in your shoes, and do not wear synthetic shoes.
- Change shoes twice or more a day. If you have to stand a lot, vary heel heights. This relieves friction and pressure points, and reduces leg fatigue. Go barefoot as much as possible; feet need air and space — they were born to be free.

- Cut toenails properly — straight across and not ultra-short — to prevent ingrowing nails. **Never** cut down the sides, or the nail grows into the skin, painfully and with risk of infection. Ill-fitting shoes can cause ingrowing nails, too. If it happens, see a chiropodist.
- Inspect feet regularly and nip foot problems in the bud or you may end up needing foot surgery. If ever you can't reach your feet, say in late pregnancy or older years, regular salon pedicures or chiropodist sessions are not treats but necessities.

Your step-by-step pedicure plan

Toenails have the same structure as fingernails, except they're thicker and grow more slowly. You need the same products and tools as for a manicure, plus: **toenail clippers** (stronger than nail scissors) and **pumice stone**, **callus file** or **skin-peeling liquid** to remove hard, dry skin.

Step 1

Scrub feet with nail brush in the bath, or in a basin of warm water. This cleans and softens the thick nails and hardened skin so you can work on them. Remove old toenail enamel as for manicure. Clip nails as described above; smooth the edges with the fine side of an emery board.

Step 2

Pumice or scrape any hard skin, or follow directions for skin peeler.

Step 3

Tend cuticles, exactly as for manicure Step 3.

Step 4

Rinse, massage in foot cream or hand/body lotion; wipe nails with enamel remover if you plan to put polish on toenails.

Step 5

Buff or proceed with coloured nail enamel exactly as for fingernails. Tiny toenails may need only a single-stroke application. Use folded tissues or a specially shaped sponge to separate toes while polish layers dry.

Sleek and silky: skin all over

Product lowdown: bath and body hygiene

In general, it's best to use **normal bath soap** (today's soaps are actually mild, non-soap detergents). Avoid deodorising soaps which can interfere with the re-establishment of the healthy bacteria that live on the skin and fight infection.

Though luxurious fun, bubble baths and bath/shower gels are detergents which can dry out or irritate the skin. So can bath crystals and salts which scent and soften the water. However, **bath milks**, that are actually made with milk, soften without harshness, and **aromatherapy oils** and **herb bags** generally have safe, soothing properties. **Bath oils** (in bottles or colourful individual capsules) are good for dryness; they moisturise by coating the skin with a fine oily film but they leave a film on the bath, too, alas! Be aware of your body skin and if it's dry, itchy or tending to rashes, switch away from bath additives for a while.

Body lotion need not be a separate extra purchase. All moisturising lotions work in the same basic way (see 'Product lowdown', Chapter 4) – you could use just one basic moisturiser for face, hands, arms and everywhere else. However, most people prefer various scents and consistencies for various purposes. A body lotion with a luscious fragrance is a delight.

Underarm deodorants stop bacteria from breaking down perspiration (which releases odour); **antiperspirants** actually stop perspiration by dehydrating sweat glands (the sweat is diverted elsewhere). **Roll-on** or **stick** formulae put the product exactly where you want it; **sprays** are easy to use and dry quickly. If you develop irritated skin, change brands; don't use antiperspirant or deodorant on broken skin or immediately after shaving your armpits.

Feminine deodorants, washes, etc. are unnecessary and potentially risky because their ingredients can interfere with natural vaginal cleansing processes. Regular bathing with simple soap and water is sufficient. Unpleasant vaginal odour or discharges are signs of infection – see your doctor. See Chapter 10.

Specific body problem areas

Focus on thighs: the great cellulite debate

For years doctors said cellulite didn't exist, perhaps because it is no medical emergency. Now most beauty experts make a convincing scientific case for cellulite and its treatment. It shows up as lumpy 'orange peel', 'cottage cheese' or puckered 'mattress' skin on the thighs. The cause is said to be fat cells which compress surrounding tissue, resulting in poor lymph and blood circulation, water retention and consequent toughening of protein fibres deep in skin. Poor exercise is implicated, so are toxins (due to tea, coffee, alcohol, refined foods), so are hormones and the very nature of fatty cells. Prime cellulite sites are thighs, hips, bottom, and the fleshy upper arm. Normal diet and exercise can't release the trapped fluid and fat.

What to do? You can just accept it as a fact of womanhood – women have more fatty cells than men, more strategically concentrated below the waist. Or you can try to prevent it in the first place by a healthy diet and good exercise. If it creeps up and concerns you, you can try one of the **anti-cellulite creams**, but be fully aware that the chief success ingredient in these is the massaging you do to rub them in. Thorough, close massage is the secret of shifting those protein fibres to release trapped fluids and improve circulation (you still need good diet and exercise to deal with fat). Count on a 14- to 30-day course before you can measure results.

Salons offer a range of cellulite beaters (**creams**, **body masks**, **body wraps**, **mild electrical stimulation**, **professional massage**, **pressure treatment**) and there are a few medical solutions involving local skin treatment. They work on lymphatic drainage and muscle toning, along the same principle as massage-in creams. With some you can measure small instant improvement, although a course of sessions gives best results. The effect won't be permanent, however, without good diet and health routines.

Focus on the bust: can it grow?

Breast enlargement by vacuum suction or firming by specialist creams is strictly fantasy, although creams or gels can moisturise the skin.

The best breast improver and maintainer is a properly-fitting bra. Always be breast aware: show lumps, puckers or skin changes to your doctor. If you are seriously unhappy with your bust, see Chapter 11.

Focus on body hair: making it disappear

A downy, fair fuzz can look delightful, but most women don't want long, dark, body hair. Some cultures and traditions like the natural look of leg hair and find underarm hair sexy; the Anglo ideal of beauty calls for sleek, smooth skin in these places. The choice is yours – but if you keep underarm hair remember that perspiration odour will cling more readily, so use spray deodorant/antiperspirant fastidiously.

Some hair-removal methods are better to use on one part of the body than another. Some methods are easier, some last longer, some cost less than others. Whatever the method, for large areas always use moisturiser afterwards, and for underarms do not use antiperspirant/deodorant for at least two hours afterwards.

Bleaching

Bleaching is ideal for soft arm hair if yours is excessive and dark. It is also good for facial hair on the upper lip or chin. Buy a special bleach for this delicate work; never use normal hair-bleaching products. Always do a skin-patch test before you proceed.

Shaving

Shaving is a popular method for legs, underarms and bikini area because it's so quick, easy and cheap. Use shaving cream on wet skin for the best finish. *Drawbacks*: occasional razor knicks and blunt hair ends. Instead of a natural, tapered regrowth, hair regrows, looking thick and feeling stubbly. The solution is to shave frequently, say once a week. Because of the stubble factor you should never shave facial hair.

Depilatory

Excellent for all areas (except eyebrows), depilatories come as creams, gels or sprays. They contain a chemical such as calcium thioglycollate which dissolves surface hair. You get smoother, longer-lasting results (about ten days) than shaving because the hair is removed slightly below the surface and the regrowth isn't blunt. *Drawbacks:* messy to use and smell strong – you have to wait five minutes or so as the chemical works, then wipe away cream and hairs. There's risk of skin irritation – this is powerful stuff, so you must do a skin-patch test first.

Plucking

Perfect for those odd sprouts of hair around nipples and tummy, and for eyebrows and other facial hair (see Chapter 3). Use tweezers to pull out one hair at a time in the direction of growth – the root comes out too. Hair regrowth is slow, soft and tapered. *Drawbacks:* it's a bit painful, and far too tedious for large areas. Threading, a skill practised in Mediterranean and Asian cultures, twists a cotton thread over skin and pulls out hairs by the roots, similar to plucking.

Waxing

Suitable for any part of the body, most often used for legs and bikini area, waxing provides really smooth, longest-lasting results because hairs are pulled out by the roots. Regrowth shows in about four weeks, and it's soft and tapered. Home waxing, with strips of cold wax, isn't as effective as salon hot or warm waxing. *Drawbacks:* it's more expensive than other methods, and it's painful; skin may be irritated for a day afterwards. Also, hair has to regrow to about 0.5 mm (¼inch) before wax can coat and grip the hairs to pull them out. Sugaring, practised in the Middle East, uses a caramel of sugar, water and lemon juice to pull hairs away, like the waxing process.

Electrolysis

Expensive, time-consuming and painful, electrolysis is really most suitable for facial hair, but you could consider it for other small areas. Its big advantage is that the removal is permanent. Only a professional can do electrolysis (see Chapter 11).

Tan fantastic

Fantastically stupid, that's what a tan is. It's nature's imperfect way of protecting you from burning sun rays. Even ordinary winter daylight damages the skin; obviously, hours under a high summer sun is worse. Today, over 40,000 people a year in the UK develop skin cancer, but somehow a tan remains appealing to most people. If you will insist on tanning, you should know the facts, and know the limits.

How skin tanning works

Normal skin colour comes from melanin, natural pigment produced by melanocytes in the epidermis. The melanin works its way up towards the surface. Exposure to intense sun rays triggers extra melanin production. It's the body's defence against sun, a chemical process which takes 36 to 48 hours after first exposure. Fair people have relatively inactive melanocytes, which means they tan lightly and slowly. Naturally dark-skinned people and fast-tanners, including those with black, Asian and Latina heritage, have active melanocytes. Burning is *not* part of the process; you do not have to turn red before you tan.

How sun rays work

Two kinds of ultraviolet (UV) rays reach the Earth from the sun. UVA rays work on the melanin already in the epidermis; this means a rapid tan for people with active melanocytes. UVA rays also damage the protein fibres (collagen, elastin, reticulin) which give skin its firmness and suppleness; this means ageing.

UVB rays penetrate melanocytes themselves, making them produce more melanin; the pigmentation takes longer to appear than the UVA stimulus, but it stays longer. UVB rays also thicken the epidermis, burn the skin and cause skin cancer.

Both kinds of rays bombard us all year round, but they are more intense in summer months, in the hours from 11 a.m. to 3 p.m., and nearer to the equator. They are also intensified by reflection off water, sand, snow, white surfaces. Sun rays also transmit heat, which robs skin of moisture, promoting dryness and lines.

How sunscreens work

There are two methods of sunscreening. **Physical sunscreens** use particles to reflect UV rays; it takes some effort to rub them into the skin. Some are **total sunblocks**. **Chemical sunscreens** use chemicals to absorb UV rays once they penetrate the skin; the tanning effect is filtered. UVA (tanning and ageing) protection as yet has no agreed rating system, and not all products offer it. The amount of UVB (tanning, burning, cancer) protection is rated by an SPF (Sun Protection Factor) from 2 to 30 or so. For this you need to know your skin tanning type, because the number means that you can stay in the sun for twice as long (SPF2) or 10 times as long (SPF10), etc, as you normally would before burning. There's a limit, however – SPF15 gives 93 per cent protection, but SPF34 gives only 97 per cent.

Always put on sunscreens 15 to 30 minutes before exposure to the sun (they take that long to penetrate). Be patient; you can't rush your skin-tanning type: 45 minutes protected exposure is all the stimulation your melanocytes can use in one day. It takes two days for the melanin to show up.

For the smoothest holiday tan (if you must tan) exfoliate skin the week before sun exposure, moisturise generously after every sun exposure. **After-sun lotions** contain cooling, soothing ingredients, but any body lotion will do. To protect hair colour in sunny climes use special **hair products with added sunscreens**.

What about non-sun tans?

Sunbeds

Sunbeds are no safer and no faster than the sun's UVA and UVB rays. Follow the same tanning limits; do not try to rush the process. If you must, sunbed to start a tan before a holiday or extend it afterwards, or to help oily skin troubles, but don't attempt a year-round tan – do you really want skin like leather and constant fear of cancer?

Self-tanning lotions

These contain a petrochemical called dihydroxyacetone which reacts harmlessly with the keratin in the skin, gradually (over two to three hours) producing a yellow-brown colour. For natural, even results exfoliate before application – follow manufacturers' instructions. The fake tan lasts for a few days until skin cells shed. Use self-tanners to fill in strap marks, to fake or to prolong a tan.

Bronzing gels

These are available under a variety of names – possibly also powders. They are translucent tints that give you the look of a tan for a day or evening, then cleanse off. You can use these as you would self-tanners, and you may prefer the richer, less yellowy look.

> ### SKIN WATCH: MOLE PATROL
> Sun or no sun, something new in your skin or in moles could indicate cancer; it's usually easy to deal with **if something's done right away**. In particular, see a doctor if you notice a mole that: suddenly appears, grows, changes colour, itches, bleeds.

Five simplified top-to-toe beauty carers

1 For rough, dry skin on heels, hands, elbows – rub the area with a teaspoonful of salt mixed with a teaspoonful of sunflower oil. Alternative: sugar with oil.
2 Sunburn relief – spread yogurt or milk on tender skin to cool and soothe. Or wipe with strong, cold tea.
3 Moisturising bath – a capful of baby oil in bath water coats the skin with a fine film of oil.
4 A bath to soothe dry skin – add one pint of milk or one cup of powdered milk to bathwater.
5 Mood baths – a handful of fresh or dry herbs tied in a muslin bag; hang from the tap into the water. Or put herbal teabags in the bath.
   - *Invigorating:* rosemary, peppermint
   - *Refreshing:* lavender, lemon balm
   - *Relaxing:* rose petals, elderflowers, camomile

10

YOUR WELLSPRING OF WELLBEING: BODY, SOUL AND SELF

Your body is the place where your self lives, and this integration is a dynamic relationship that affects health, looks and confidence. Tuning into and taking care of your whole self is a simple matter of awareness and easy self-management tactics. In this chapter I start with stress, so much a part of life, and take three diversions: the immune system (because it has so much to do with wellbeing), hormones (because they have a big impact on women's health and looks) and some women's health matters (because knowledge can save you trouble, even save your life).

The chapter comes full circle with de-stressing 'how-to's essential to holistic health and beauty.

Stress survival

Stress is normal. It comes from both good things – think of the feelings involved when you receive an award, get a promotion, get married – and bad things such as fear of redundancy, illness in the family, a big tax bill. In many ways stress is a good thing: it helps to keep us alert. However, frequent surges of stress, or constant or underlying stress, wear the body down.

The stress mechanism kicks powerful forces into action. Our bodies are still biologically tuned to the wild old days when the solution was fight (the attacking sabre-toothed tiger) or flight (from the oncoming woolly mammoth). There's instant decision-making (Do I run or stand

and fight?). Hormones, particularly adrenalin, the life-booster, flood through your system. Blood is diverted towards brain and heart, away from less essential organs. Blood sugar rises for instant energy. Breathing deepens for extra oxygen. Muscles tense, ready to move. When the danger is past, shakiness and change in breath pattern are indicators that the body is returning from emergency alert to normal status.

Today when you're stressed by an on coming bus your body's reactions are still appropriate. When you're stressed by an irritating colleague or a fussy baby or by mounting bills or traffic jams or any of a million other modern-day situations, your stress mechanism works in the same old Stone Age way. However, in our situations stress is usually drip-fed instead of coming as rampaging one-offs, and you rarely get to the release-and-relief stage. You don't usually punch colleagues, walk away from babies or kill bills. There's no fight, no flight, and the stress alert doesn't shut down.

What with one stress and another, your body can be in a steady state of ready-for-action. Eventually, it's wearing.

Eventually, excess stress affects:

- wellbeing and health – chronic stress can lead to intestinal disorders, asthma, migraines, high blood pressure causing risk of heart disease, and other problems.
- personality – stress can make you tense, irritable, nagging, short tempered, moody. You may lack a sense of humour, feel you're not in control or never have enough time, lose peace of mind and confidence.
- looks – stress shows up as frown lines, skin flare-ups, undereye circles and 'grey' skin from insomnia. You may overeat, drink alcohol or smoke to relieve stress, affecting your weight, skin and wellbeing.

Stress isn't all bad, however. What's stressful to one person doesn't faze another. And life itself is stress; without stress your life would be a bland and boring safety zone – even boredom is stressful. The trick is to learn to de-stress yourself; it's easy when you know how.

There are two main routes to stress recovery: the body and the mind. There is more to come on this later in this chapter, but first a health-wise diversion in which stress is strongly involved.

A system to beat illness and toxins

In beauty massage, facials and electric-technology assisted body treatments, salons and clinics often talk about **lymphatic drainage**. Just what is it? A lot more than a beauty booster (details on that aspect in a moment), the lymphatic system is an integral part of the immune system.

A strong immune system keeps you healthy, a weak one makes you susceptible to viruses, cycles of thrush or herpes, and other more serious nasties. In peak form it protects you from infection by bacteria, viruses, fungi, even cancer. It's an amazing and complex mini-universe which you have some inkling about if you know of polio vaccine, measles immunisation or HIV and AIDS.

You can take care of your immune system, so it can take care of you. Its warriors and scavengers are transported through the body by the blood and by a related liquid called **lymph**. For the general purpose of staying healthy and looking good you need to know about this key element.

The focus here is microcirculation, the cardio-vascular system at its most distant point: a plasma-like tissue fluid that bathes every cell in the body. This tissue fluid filters through the tiniest blood capillaries to reach body cells, carrying nourishment (see 'Cell power', Chapter 1). On the return journey, carrying waste, some tissue fluid passes into lymph capillaries – at which point it's called lymph. The network of lymph vessels eventually pours the fluid back into the bloodstream, but along the way it passes through lymph nodes clustered in various places around the body.

Here's where the lymphatic system makes its huge contribution to your immunity. Locally, nodes fight infection; for instance, they're at work if you can feel enlarged nodes ('swollen glands') in your neck below your ear when you have a sore throat. But lymph tissue also works widely, for it forms antibodies and it houses special white blood cells and releases them into the circulation to fight infection throughout your body.

One more thing about the lymphatic system – and this directly affects your good looks: without a heart to power it, lymph circulation relies mainly on the movement of the body's muscles, helped by exertion or pressure. If lymph drainage is sluggish the result is the puffiness we call water retention; toxins as well as water are trapped in the tissue area. This most commonly occurs in feet, ankles, abdomen and eye area.

What can you do to support your immune system for wellbeing and good looks?

- Indulge in massage – it can speed up the rate of lymphatic drainage and release stress.
- Release stress – chronic stress depresses the immune system (you will find de-stress hints at the end of this chapter).
- Enjoy a healthy eating and exercise lifestyle – the immune system needs nutrients and oxygen.

Ages and stages: hormones, health and looks

Hormones are chemicals released in one part of the body to circulate in the blood and act on another part. Working in intricate harmony, hormones control numerous body functions including cell metabolism, response to stress or illness (recall adrenalin in the fight or flight mechanism?), growth and sexual development.

It's this last area that's particularly relevant to your looks and sense of wellbeing. In women, the ovaries produce the hormones oestrogen and progesterone in varied amounts at different stages of life – to powerful effect. They can wreak havoc with your life and looks, though they also bring about great sexy feelings and good moods.

Teen upheavals – 11 to 18 years

Beginning as early as age ten oestrogen levels increase, starting the development of breasts, the growth of pubic and underarm hair, the widening of hips, and uterus enlargement. Height and weight increase, too, and at some point the first menstrual period occurs. The whole process takes about four years, and it's a huge upheaval for the body and the girl living through this surge towards adult womanhood.

Looks-wise, the hormones cause an increase of oils in skin and hair – bad enough in itself to be shiny and greasy, worse when the oil excess leads to pimples, blackheads or acne. Hair may change character, thickening, darkening, acting up; leg hairs may grow longer and darker; underarm hair traps perspiration which is now stronger-smelling. Chapters 4 to 9 are full of advice on how to handle these new challenges.

On top of your physiological changes, you have to get used to your new breasts, larger feet, changing shape, and the hormones contribute to swings of mood, so sometimes you feel life's great, and at other times you want to bury yourself in a blanket. Your relationships with girl and boy friends and parents, and your feelings about the future and the universe change, waver and develop in these years. Good health and beauty self-care is a natural way to help yourself cope.

Fertile cycles – 18 to 45 years

Oestrogen has the upper hand in the first half of your menstrual cycle; progesterone steps up after ovulation (release of an egg by an ovary). If the egg isn't fertilised and pregnancy doesn't happen, the progesterone slackens off. This regular cycle – anything from 24 to 35 days including the bloodshedding period of about 5 days – ideally goes as smoothly as clockwork.

However, many women have some sign of the hormonal swings, usually pimples, as the period approaches. And many at some time have premenstrual syndrome (PMS) with physical symptoms of breast tenderness, fluid retention, headache, backache and emotional symptoms (sometimes called PMT, where T is for tension) of irritability, depression, fatigue. In addition, some women have minor or severe pain at the time of their periods, usually cramps. The hormonal cycles can be disrupted, too, by intense stress, illness or excessive physical training or weight loss – periods come at random times or don't come at all.

Of course all this fertility is meant to make babies, so contraception is an issue, and a choice you make. It can conveniently make use of oestrogen and/or progestogen (synthetic progesterone) with the contraceptive pill, mini-pill, injections or implants. Other methods (coil, condom, diaphragm with spermicide, sterilisation) physically prevent fertilisation. The rhythm method, which means no unprotected sex in the fertile days, relies on a predictable cycle. These all have advantages and disadvantages, but only the hormone-based methods tend to cause weight gain and other PMS-type side effects.

The downside effects of fertile womanhood may not do much for your feelgood factor or your looks. The best antidote is to keep a brief, daily diary throughout two cycles so you can see patterns emerge. You can, then, at least be forewarned about low days and nurture yourself through them instead of being just a victim.

Contraception – the coil or pill – may need changing; it can aggravate or improve period problems. Progesterone supplements may help. Look into other remedies – vitamin supplements, evening primrose oil, diet, vitamin B6, stress reduction. See the complementary medicine section later in this chapter.

Interludes – pregnancy and childbirth

Pregnancy is a mega-hormonal time as your body nourishes and supports the developing baby. Many women feel marvellously happy and calm through most of the pregnancy – one of progesterone's side effects. There is also a downside for many: morning sickness, tiredness, indigestion, possibly haemorrhoids and varicose veins. Besides the obvious visible effects of breast enlargement and an ever-growing bump, pregnancy has other impacts on your looks.

- Hair is usually lush and thick, although in some women it thins.
- Skin may have a wonderful creamy glow, although some get greasy skin and spots. Women with dry skin may find it gets even drier, tight and itchy all over the body.
- Well into pregnancy the characteristic butterfly-shaped mask – a freckle-coloured pigmentation – may appear; it spreads from nose over cheeks and sometimes forehead. It can be quite attractive, like extra blusher, though it fades after the baby is born. Other pigment changes include a darkened nipple area and a dark line from navel to pubic hair.
- Stretch marks may show up on breasts or abdomen. Red at first, they are caused when elastic fibres beneath the skin surface have overstretched and ruptured. After birth, breast stretch marks fade to thin, silvery lines and they usually disappear after breastfeeding. Abdominal stretch marks may not occur if weight gain is less than 9 kg (20 lb); they fade eventually, too, but not entirely.

These are all proud marks of pregnancy, so why not enjoy flaunting them? Good skincare, haircare and bodycare will help you through, and attention to make-up and hairstyling can help you feel smart as your bump burgeons. Early days with the new baby are so fulfilling and demanding that you may have little time for attention to yourself. By about six weeks, though, you can begin exercise (doctor's advice permitting), not only for vanity but to get abdominal and pelvic muscles strong again (See 'Exercise your sex muscle' in Chapter 3). It may take a bit longer before you feel you can tear yourself away for a haircut.

Changes – 45 to 55 years and beyond

Starting in the early forties some periods may occur without an egg having been released. This upsets the hormones, and therefore the rhythm of menstruation – periods may be longer, shorter, late, frequent; PMS may occur for the first time. Changes like these signal the start of perimenopause (around the menopause), a lead-up to the menopause (cessation of menstruation). Like the kicking-in of fertility in adolescence, the changeover takes four or five years, and like the teen years it can be a time of physical and psychological upheaval.

Some women have no menopausal troubles at all, many have hot flushes and night sweats, some have vaginal dryness that makes intercourse difficult. Decreasing hormone levels affect looks, too: skin gets drier and begins to lose plumpness and elasticity, hair thins, may go grey, may change behaviour, and hairs may sprout at chin or upper lip. As if these changes aren't enough, other common symptoms are poor concentration, depression, anxiety and loss of interest in sex.

All of this can add up to plummeting confidence, and it can come just as your children are turning into grown-ups and/or your career horizons change. Much like a teenager, you move from the known to the unknown, adapting your attitudes to friends, family, life and the universe.

To ease you through, try a super-healthy diet and lifestyle, and possibly evening primrose oil, B vitamins and other supplements. Hormone replacement therapy (HRT) resolves many of the menopausal symptoms, although some women don't like its side effects. On HRT you will probably continue to get a period (unless you've had a hysterectomy). Some women get help from progesterone cream alone, applied to the skin, or oestrogen cream for vaginal dryness.

Adjustments in skin, hair and body routines are called for. Make-up palette and hairstyle or colour, clothes' colours too, may need revising. Massages can help both physically and psychologically.

YOUR WELLSPRING OF WELLBEING: BODY, SOUL AND SELF

By age 55 you should be there – free of periods, in your stride and full of energy in this third stage of womanhood. There's a further hormonal kickback, however: the lack of hormones may cause osteoporosis and atherosclerosis, risks to your health. The first is the bone thinning, bone brittling that eventually leads to 'old people's' bone breaks. The second is narrowing of arteries by fatty deposits that can increase the chance of heart disease and stroke. Correct diet, possibly with nutritional supplements, and bone-pounding, weight-bearing exercise can keep these at bay. For some women HRT or progesterone cream is the way to prevent them.

Women's health matters

Eleven easy ways to save a woman's life

A diary and a doctor can save you from life-destroying diseases. Many listed on the next page are common only to women; all can be avoided, cured or safely managed if detected in time. Besides a general health check-up every five years or so (annually from age 75), have the screening checks on schedule, as indicated (points 1 to 4), ask for others (points 5 to 9) if you have reason for suspicion. The last two lifesaving points (10 and 11) are sheer common sense.

Two plagues on women, plus a risk

Thrush

Three out of four women get this vaginal condition at some point in their lives. Symptoms may include itching, soreness, stinging on urination, painful sexual intercourse, and a discharge (not the light discharge of normal health but a thick, curdy, white discharge that's not particularly smelly).

It's caused by *Candida albicans*, a yeast living in the body that's normally kept under control by the immune system. Factors that can throw out this normal balance: being stressed, run-down, pregnant, on the contraceptive pill or antibiotics. See a doctor to confirm that it's thrush; it's cured by creams, pessaries or a capsule by mouth.

What	Why?	When?
1 Cervical smear	Cervical cancer	Every 3–5 years from age 20 or age of first sexual activity.
2 Breast awareness	Breast cancer	Show any changes to your doctor. Mammogram for women aged 50–64 every 3 years.
3 Blood pressure	Heart disease, stroke, kidneys	Every 4 years until age 40, then every 2 years or annually if on oral contraceptive pill.
4 Vision	Glaucoma blindness	Every 2 years, from age 40.
5 Blood sugar	Diabetes	From age 40 as part of general check-up.
6 Blood cholesterol	Heart disease	Any age, if high blood pressure or family heart disease history.
7 Blood sex-hormones	Menopausal symptoms, osteoporosis, thyroid	Any age if menopausal symptoms; from 50 if unexplained weight loss or lethargy
8 Bone density	Osteoporosis	If blood sex-hormones, family history or menopause suggest.
9 Ovarian scan	Ovarian cancer	If family history, or childless and over age 50.
10 Don't smoke	Heart disease, stroke, lung cancer, diabetes, cervical cancer	All ages.
11 No unprotected sex	HIV/AIDS, other sexually-transmitted diseases, cervical cancer	All ages.

Preventive helps:

- Wear loose-fitting skirts and trousers, cotton gusseted underwear and tights to allow air circulation.
- Wipe from front to back after a bowel movement to avoid carrying the yeast from the bowel.
- Avoid bath additives, perfumed soaps, vaginal deodorants, douches. They can irritate and upset the natural balance of the vagina.

Cystitis

Most women have cystitis at some time, and men hardly ever do. It's not fair, but it's because women's urethras (tube from bladder to urine outlet) are short. Germs find it easy to travel up the urethra to the bladder itself and cause an inflammation. The result: frequent need to pass urine, but only small amounts accompanied by burning, stinging pain.

See a doctor to check if you need antibiotics. But even before you do that, start drinking copious amounts of water to help flush out the bladder, and try to empty the bladder completely each time you pass water. Keep urine alkaline (to ease the irritation) by taking a teaspoon of sodium bicarbonate in water every six hours.

Preventive helps:

Same as for thrush, plus one more:
- if you're prone to cystitis, pass water as soon as you can after making love.

Toxic Shock Syndrome (TSS)

This is a rare condition of massive life-threatening blood poisoning. For unknown reasons young women aged 16 to 26 are more at risk than others when wearing tampons during their periods. Each year one or two women die, perhaps eight more are severely ill. The first symptoms are flu-like, so if you're using a tampon and come down with a high temperature (139 °C/102 °F), aches, sore throat, etc. remove the tampon and see your doctor or emergency clinic at once: rapid and huge doses of antibiotics are needed.

Preventive helps:

TSS is rare, so don't panic, but do:
- wash hands before and after changing tampons
- change tampons every four to six hours
- use minimum absorbency for your flow.

Your own de-stress plan

Stress relief: the body path

The stress mechanism causes muscle tension. Let go of muscle tension regularly and the body bounces (or drifts) back to recovery. Try to release stress physically every day, or at least every other day, by some of the methods below.

Action release Any of the aerobic exercises, weight workouts, and many of the active stretches in Chapter 3 are effective for action release.

Relaxation release You can use all of the slow stretches in Chapter 3. The Complete Yoga Breath (p. 35) is effective and easy; do it during busy days, at stressed moments, any time, anywhere. It's also great for getting you calm just before bed for a good night's sleep, another key de-stressor. Another route is via a gym or beauty clinic sauna or whirlpool; the heat or swirl unwinds muscles.

Touch release Hands-on massage works the kinks out, stimulating lymph drainage and energy flow. You may not know what real relaxation feels like until a professional works her or his magic. A bonus: the feeling of being nurtured contributes to emotional tension release. Go to a gym, beauty clinic or salon for a body massage, aromatherapy, facial, manicure or pedicure. You can also massage yourself.

Do-it-yourself facial massage
The face is a great storer of tension but also a great gateway to restoring calm. At the start or end of the day, or as often as you need, massage your face with some or all of these shiatsu techniques – see illustration. Use the tips of your middle and first fingers, middle finger to press firmly on the specific points for three to five seconds. Repeat each action three times.

1 Stroke up from the neck and over cheeks. Then from centre of forehead to temples. Press temple points.

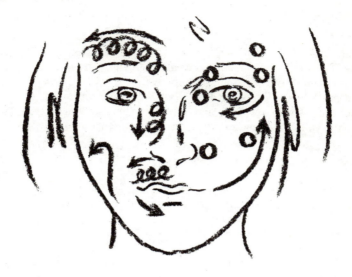

Figure 13 Do-it-yourself facial massage for stress and skin microcirculation.

2 Gently drum forehead from centre to temples. Make gentle corkscrew-like circles along eyebrows from nose to temple. Lightly stroke under eye to inner corner. Press inner brow points, then end-of-brow points.
3 Press points either side of bridge of nose. Lightly corkscrew down sides of nose to lower nostril points. Press.
4 Corkscrew over lips from centre to corners. Lightly sweep under mouth. Make swirling motions gently from mouth corners up to ears. Press points under cheekbones.

Hand pinch
Another quick shiatsu de-stressor is the hand pinch. Using one hand, place your thumb above, fingers beneath the fleshiest part of the V between the bones of the thumb and index finger of the other hand. Press down hard with the thumb for seven to ten seconds. Release and repeat, reversing hands.

Complementary medicine release Hands-on treatments can release general body tensions. Try Alexander Technique, osteopathy, acupuncture, shiatsu massage, reflexology (see section later in this chapter).

Intake release Coffee, tea and cola give you a lift because of their caffeine. Tranquillisers, smoking and alcohol calm you down, but regular use is harmful. Cut back on stressors, eat for peace – review Chapter 2. For times of extra stress or after illness, consider vitamin and mineral supplements with extra C and B-complex, possibly Korean ginseng, plenty of calming herbal teas: camomile, limeflower, lemon balm.

Stress relief: the mind path

Mind, here, includes emotions, attitudes, lifestyle and values. Every day, give a thought to your activities and your interactions with other people and the world around you, and try some of the stress-relieving, calm-inducing methods below.

Paper relief Make a list of all the things you have to do when you're buzzing with stress. Pick out the three biggest 'musts' and one purely 'I want to'; let the rest wait until tomorrow. Keep a daily diary briefly noting your stressed times; review in six weeks to see if a pattern emerges, maybe PMT, food allergy, or another culprit you can deal with. Or keep an intermittant journal, a place to write freely and privately, pouring out feelings and observations.

People relief This may mean time out from people – letting the answering machine take calls, going out for a walk alone, lingering in the bath, sneaking ten minutes of peace before you return to home or work. It can also mean phoning a friend or relative for a good moan or gossip, making time for social get-togethers, cuddling your kids or your lover.

Mind relief A relaxed mind refreshes and relaxes the whole body. Meditation can involve just concentrating on a simple occupation (gardening, needlepoint, knitting, pottery, jogging – it should be absorbing, solitary and physically repetitive). You might want to learn to meditate by going to a class; Transcendental Meditation (TM) is proven as a de-stressor. Guided imagery, learned from classes or self-help books (such as *Teach Yourself Visualisation* in this series), is another delightful mental route to relaxation.

Stress trigger relief List things that cause you stress. When they occur (traffic jams, screaming child) be aware of your body tensions and consciously de-tense – you can do Complete Yoga Breath (p. 35), lion face (p.35), chest expansion (p. 55) quickly and not too obviously. Try to figure out stress situations you can change (leave for work earlier? anticipate and defuse the child's stress?). For those you can't (noisy aeroplanes, a broken leg) try to change your own attitude.

Perspective relief Dwell now and then on your place – and stresses – in the scheme of things. Is the problem really so earth-shaking? Personal growth and spiritual development through religion, classes or reading can help this. So can awareness of – even voluntary work for – the oppressed, poor, ill or disabled, or another cause. Take an overview of your own life, too: look back on yourself five years ago, look ahead five years. Count your blessings.

Pleasure relief The smell of fresh flowers, the touch of warm sun, the sweep of a concerto, a chocolate truffle, vintage red wine – consciously savour the sensual pleasures of life, without a guilt attack; some doctors now worry that 'healthism' undermines wellbeing. Medical science says lovemaking mingles mind and body paths for ideal stress relief, actually releasing endorphins, feelgood brain chemicals; a nice bonus is that it also does good things for your relationship. Other pleasure relationships count, too. Stroke the cat, walk the dog, watch the goldfish. Play with kids (roughhouse, fingerpaint, shout for echoes, dance). Get totally giggly with friends or family. Go the other way and have a good cry. Laughter, tears and smiles, like love, release de-stressing brain chemicals.

Body and self wellbeing

Complementary medicine for healthy beauty

For your looks and for stress, hormonal upheavals, chronic conditions or minor illnesses, complementary medicine could be the answer, especially when you've found no relief from conventional medicine. As well as helping problems such as asthma, backache, indigestion, hayfever, migraine, PMT, etc., they can tune up your immune system and generally stimulate your energy and confidence. Benefits often include better skin, posture and metabolism.

Choose a therapy that appeals to you – acupuncture, Alexander Technique, chiropractice or osteopathy, herbalism, homoeopathy, reflexology, shiatsu, others. Find a practitioner by word of mouth, through a natural health clinic or a national organisation. (See Resources at back of this book.) Always be sure the practitioner you choose is a certified member of her or his discipline's professional body. You usually need three to a dozen sessions over one to six months, depending on the problem and the therapy. If you feel no improvement by six weeks, it's probably not the right therapy for you.

WELLBEING WOBBLIES

So, life's not perfect. It happens. Here are some rescues.

Insomnia A mug of warm milk, perhaps sprinkled with cinnamon. Complete Yoga Breaths. Imagining a fantasy world.

Colds and 'flu A hot toddy: a mug of hot water with a big dash of lemon juice, a teaspoon of sugar or honey, stir in a dash of whisky for warmth and comfort. Take herbal echinacea or garlic to build up immune system.

Sore throat or blocked nose Steam your face over a bowl of hot water containing a few camomile teabags to soothe a throat, or two tablespoons of thyme for nose.

Indigestion Drink peppermint tea. Or try homoeopathic remedies carbo veg or nux vom. Fast on fruit and vegetables for a day.

Hangover Plenty of water (ideally before bed, too), fruit juices, vitamins B and C, evening primrose oil. Painkillers for headache.

Jet lag Set your watch to destination time as soon as you take off. Drink lots of water and no alcohol in flight. Nap or early to bed on arrival. Try melatonin, the 'body clock hormone', to aid sleep patterns.

Feeling blue or stressed Pinch fresh or dried lavender flowers and inhale the aroma.

11
PROFESSIONAL AND MEDICAL BEAUTY INTERVENTION

So, you do everything possible – cleanse, tone, eat the right foods, follow the right lifestyle, develop your personal style, make the most of make-up and hair – and you're still not satisfied? Maybe you're thinking about taking an irrevocable step, a permanent change in your looks that involves a licensed professional. Could be better teeth, a tattoo, a face lift: some changes are fairly easy to achieve, some are for fun, others are serious stuff. It's okay: you are allowed to do it. It's *your* body, *your* self, *your* looks. But of course you need to think clearly before you decide. The three major issues are sorting out *why* you want this change, understanding just *what* is involved in this kind of intervention, and finding the practitioner *who* is qualified. Cost is a consideration, too.

A beautiful smile: cosmetic dentistry

All smiles are beautiful, but perhaps the look of your teeth stops you from smiling as often as you could? Cosmetic dental improvements can be surprisingly easy and satisfying. See sections later in this chapter on making your decision and finding who'll do it; below is an idea of what can be done.

Chips, gaps, uneven, short or too-pointy teeth

These can often be corrected with amazing ease and at very reasonable expense.

Slightly uneven teeth can be simply and quickly filed into smoothness in a single visit.

Moulding allows the dentist to sculpt a putty-like resin composite to correct a problem. He or she sets the tooth-coloured material to tooth-hardness by shining a special light on it. This is the same material that is now used to give cavities 'white' instead of 'silver' fillings. A cosmetic moulding correction of one or two teeth takes only a single appointment.

Veneers cover up or fill in front-teeth flaws. Alone, they look like false fingernails because they are so wafer thin. But when the individually tailored porcelain veneers are permanently bonded on to your own teeth they look and feel quite natural and perfect. Veneers usually require two visits – one to fit and one to fix in place.

Discoloured teeth can be covered by veneers or lightened by bleach. For the latter, the surface is painted with a chemical and exposed to ultraviolet light.

Heavily filled, unsightly or missing teeth

Any of the above may be beyond the scope of veneers or moulding. However, they can be covered or replaced. These methods take some trouble and expense, but the improvement can be dramatically worth it.

Crowns and **caps** provide tooth-shaped porcelain jackets for teeth. The tooth underneath has to be filed to a pyramid shape (under local anaesthetic) so the cover-up fits perfectly. In the two weeks while the crown is being made you won't go around looking like a vampire; the dentist makes you a temporary plastic crown which looks just fine. New stronger, light-refractory materials make the real crown look and feel totally natural.

Bridges replace a missing tooth by crowning the teeth on either side of the gap and holding an additional substitute tooth between them.

Implants can replace one, several or a complete set of teeth. They take considerable time, trouble and cost, but the result is permanent, virtually natural teeth. Oral surgery by a specialist (implantologist) places a fixture in the jawbone. Thankfully this has to be done under anaesthetic, and then it takes four to six months for the implant to bond with the bone. In the final stage, natural-looking teeth are attached to the implant.

Crooked, overcrowded, widely spaced, protruding or concave teeth

If your teeth are unsuitable for the solutions above you may need **braces** – and it's never too late; any age can benefit from braces. The straightening process takes two years. It's costly but basically painless, although it requires monthly visits to the orthodontist for adjustments to the appliances that guide teeth into the correct position. The worst defects are visibly improved within the first few months. As a teen, being a 'metal mouth' has become a sort of status symbol and rite of passage. As an adult, you can put up with the silvery wires knowing that people will admire your bravery, and prizing the unselfconscious smile you'll have at the end.

Ages and stages of teeth

Many people aged 18 to 25 neglect dental care. Many aged 40 to 50 suddenly find their gums in bad shape. Pregnancy tends to soften gums due to extra hormones. At these – and all – times, be extra vigilant and avoid tedious and costly repairs by regular care.

— Cosmetic surgery: the lowdown —

Sometimes nature deals a wild card – a big mole where you don't want it, lumpy veins that shout, acne and its telltale scars. Sometimes nature is too generous or too skimpy – bust, nose, chin or another feature may make you self-conscious. Always, time marches on, leaving its marks. Is cosmetic medical treatment the answer for you? You must quiz yourself closely as to what you expect from it – more on this later in this chapter – but first, know the facts.

Birthmarks, moles, spider naevus, thread veins, skin tags, cysts

Most skin blemishes can be removed quickly and easily by minor outpatient surgery under local anaesthetic. You may need a stitch or two, to be removed a week later. Sometimes instead of surgery the blemish can be 'frozen' off, chemically, or removed or faded with laser treatment. Another alternative seals off tiny veins by injection or diathermy (like electrolysis, it delivers electric current via a fine needle); this method may take three or four short visits.

Varicose veins

If support hose are no longer the answer, surgery can remove or sclerotherapy can seal off the large, bumpy, sometimes aching veins so common on the backs and inner sides of legs. The treatment may be under general anaesthetic in hospital on an outpatient basis, or local anaesthetic in a clinic. The incisions are tiny, but you must wear a pressure bandage on the leg for a week or more afterwards. The deep vein system in the legs will do all the work that these superficial veins did.

Acne scarring

Once acne outbreaks have stopped you can smooth out the bumps and pits that remain via chemical face peeling (see below) or dermabrasion. In this, your skin is numbed with local anaesthetic and the surface is 'sanded' away by a high-speed spinning abrasive wheel. Healing takes two weeks or so, and skin will be red or pink until the final new complexion develops over a further six weeks.

Face lines and wrinkles; acne scarring

A non-surgical procedure called face peeling 'erases' the skin surface and creates a smooth, radiant complexion. It requires a one-week stay in a clinic or nursing home. Under sedation, your face is painted with a special chemical which penetrates to the dermis layer of skin and removes the top layers of the epidermis. Your face is then bandaged for two days, after which frequent facial showers help the process. By the time you are free to go home your skin will look fresh and quite pink, as if you had been sunburned. It takes about five weeks for the colour to calm down and return to normal, and you must avoid exposure to the sun until completely healed.

Facial sagging and folds

The classic face lift (rhydectomy) removes excess face skin by surgery. You can have a full face lift or a half – either *upper* to correct forehead and eye area, or *lower* to tighten jawline and neck. Under general anaesthetic in a hospital the surgeon cuts skin at the hairline (for upper face) and/or behind the ear (for lower face) and undercuts the skin as far as the 'smile' crease, then pulls the skin up and back, removes the excess skin and restitches the new edge at the incision. You have to stay in hospital for one or two nights, and you'll look swollen and bruised for about two weeks. About a week after the operation you will have the stitches out. The scars are hidden, but may remain numb for months. A face lift only takes away sags. For general lines and wrinkles you might also, or instead, consider face peeling or collagen injections.

Individual smile and frown lines, crow's feet, lipstick 'bleed' lines, acne scars, and transforming lips from pinched to pout

If your skin is generally elastic and firm and the flaw you perceive is in a limited area, a collagen implant can plump out the underlying skin structure. In a series of two to five treatments a physician injects collagen just beneath the skin where it has 'collapsed', to build up and smooth out the skin. There may be some swelling, redness or bruising afterwards. Unlike silicone, collagen is a natural substance that does not migrate; it eventually disappears, metabolised by the body. The implant lasts for about one year, and can be topped up annually.

Eye bags and sags

Surgery on the eyelids under or over the eyes (blepharoplasty) can remove droopy or puffy excess skin. It is usually done under local anaesthetic in hospital on an outpatient basis. The surgeon makes the incision so that the scar will be hidden along the upper lid crease or beneath the lower lid lash line. After the operation ice packs are applied to reduce swelling and bruising. The fine stitches are removed on a return visit five to ten days later. The eye area is bruised and swollen for up to ten days, with all swelling subsiding in a month.

Large or bumpy nose

A 'nose job' (rhynoplasty) surgically alters the structure of the nose to make it proportional with the rest of the face. It usually requires general anaesthetic and a one-night hospital stay. The surgeon makes incisions inside the nose so that no scars show, and then reshapes and realigns the cartilage and bone of the nose. It's then splinted in position for ten days or so. Considerable swelling, tenderness and bruising last about two weeks. Some swelling continues and the final effect may take weeks or months to appear.

Receding or jutting chin or jawline

A surgeon can reshape your jaw or chin by removing excess tissue to reduce it, or inserting an implant to build up the structure. This requires a general anaesthetic and a hospital stay of one or two nights. The incision is usually within the mouth, so scars will not show. Jaw, neck and chin area will be swollen and bruised for about two weeks. Some swelling may continue for a while before your final profile emerges.

Protruding ears

Usually only people who wear short hair worry about sticking-out ears, but if they bother you surgical ear correction (otoplasty) can alter the cartilage to reshape the ear. It's a fairly simple procedure, usually done under local anaesthetic in hospital. The scar is hidden in the crease behind the ear. In most cases you can go home the same day, and return in two days to have the bandages removed. You need to wear bandages when you sleep at night for two more weeks.

Large, small or droopy breasts

Mammoplasty is the medical name for the surgery that can reduce, enlarge, lift or reshape breasts. General anaesthetic and a hospital stay of one or two nights is necessary.

To reduce or lift breasts: incisions are made around the nipple, in the crease below the breast and in a vertical line from nipple to crease. Excess skin and tissue are removed, and the edges stitched.

To augment breasts: the incision is made along the crease below the breast or in the armpit. An implant is inserted in a pocket behind the breast and the incision is stitched closed. The implant usually used today is a silicone bag containing soft silicone gel, saline solution or soya bean oil.

Bandages and stitches are removed a week after the operation, and the scars should fully heal in six weeks. Breast reduction or lift is very satisfying for most women. Enlargement can be, too, but internal scar tissue can form in time around the implant, making the breast harder and changing its shape – treatment by firm pressure or a minor operation may be required to correct this.

Fatty hips, thighs, abdomen, buttocks, 'pear shape', 'saddle bags', 'love handles', 'piano legs', etc.

Unshiftable spot deposits of fat can be removed by liposucton or suction lipectomy. It won't work for generally overweight or obese people and it's no substitute for diet and exercise. Generally performed in hospital, liposuction may require general anaesthetic and a one- or two-night stay, or only local anaesthetic on a day-patient basis, depending on the complexity of the job.

The procedure involves a small incision in a skin fold near the site, so scarring is minimal. The fat in the area is broken up, then sucked out. There may be considerable blood and fluid loss, so your recovery must be closely monitored. Pressure bandages or a corset must remain in place for a week, and then be worn for part of the day for another three weeks. Minor dimpling of the skin may occur. Fat can't form in that area again, but you can still get fat elsewhere.

Saggy abdomen

Fat deposits in the stomach area may be removed by liposuction, but excess loose skin can only be removed by surgery. As with breast reduction or a face lift, the skin is pulled towards the incision (at bikini line and navel), the excess cut away and the skin stitched. This is a hospital operation requiring a two-night stay. An abdominal wound always needs special attention during recovery and the healing process. Scars heal in six weeks or so; there is some risk of large scars.

Major cosmetic changes: your decision

So now you know a few hard facts about cosmetic dental and medical treatment and you can begin to consider your decision. Clearly there are risks involved in surgery; any operation, whether for health or cosmetic reasons, can go wrong. Is the benefit – that perfect nose, great breasts, ten-years-younger face – going to be worth the risks and the pain? For there is assuredly discomfort and often pain in the facial and body procedures described above. For many you'll need pain killers and sedatives. Except for dental implants, dental cosmetic work usually involves less risk and pain than cosmetic surgery.

Most women who've had cosmetic medical treatment say the first few days are seriously uncomfortable – many admit to feeling regret. Even months after, there's numbness in scar areas. But after six months or so, most are very glad they did it, regret and pain lost in the past.

People who've had major cosmetic changes also say that their friends, family and colleagues don't usually notice the change – all that pain and expense for naught? However, they say they often get comments about how generally well they look. This 'you yourself but somehow looking extra good' is the effect cosmetic medical experts aim for, *not* a radical or artificial new you. Can you live with these realities?

And both before and after the procedure, can you live with the taboos about cosmetic medical meddling? Teeth, skin blemishes and varicose veins are generally accepted as deserving of correction, but many people seem to feel it's vain and silly to change other parts of the body. If you proceed you may have to deal with hostility, curiosity or the need to harbour a secret as if you were guilty. Above all, you should feel as sure as you can about your right to make this change. Try working through this checklist if you need help to decide.

Major cosmetic changes – should you do it?

You should because

- the flaw always bothers you
- the flaw causes physical discomfort
- you have a right to correct nature's mistake
- you've taken care of yourself and your looks
- you understand it may be painful and has risks, but in the long run you think it will be worth it
- you've read about the correction, talked about it to your own doctor and the specialist who'll do it
- you've had an honest talk with someone you know who's had a similar correction
- you want your overall appearance subtly improved
- you like yourself
- you own your body
- you can afford it financially

You shouldn't because

- it will change your life
- your partner, parent or friend has asked you to
- stars and celebrities do it all the time
- you want to look better than everyone else
- afterwards you'll start exercising and giving more care to your looks and style
- you hate yourself
- you want everyone to notice you
- your friend had the same thing done
- it will save your marriage
- you want instant, dramatic change

Who will do it?

To search out a skilled and qualified professional you can:

- ask your doctor (or dentist, in the case of cosmetic dentistry) to recommend someone;
- use word-of-mouth; the experience of a friend or friend-of-a-friend is often the best path;
- contact clinics or organisations mentioned in magazine or newspaper articles, or in adverts at the back of beauty magazines;
- contact the professional association of the specialist service you seek.

Always make sure the practitioner is licensed and qualified by his or her professional body.

How to proceed?

Discuss full details of the procedure; ideally see more than one specialist before deciding. Ask:

- What happens before and during the procedure?
- How much pain will there be?
- How will I feel immediately afterwards?
- How will I look? Ask to see photos of previous clients.
- When will I feel and look my new self?
- What are the risks?
- Where will scars be (if any)?
- How permanent is the procedure?
- What if I'm not happy with the results?

Always ask to talk to a previous client; good practitioners encourage this.

How much will it cost?

Discuss costs fully. Generally, the more complex the procedure and the longer the full treatment takes, the more expensive it will be. Be sure that:

- all costs are included – no surprises at the end, like follow-up prescriptions or meal charges for a hospital stay;
- your advance payment is refundable if you change your mind – good practitioners allow this.

Permanent body decoration: piercing, tattoos, make-up

A dashing way to make a personal style statement, decorating the body by making use of the skin's own healing characteristics goes back to ancient civilisations. Something to bear in mind: in putting colour into the skin or putting holes through it you are actually wounding the skin, and, of course, the change is permanent – which is part of the daring glamour.

People and places offering these services in Britain must be registered with the local environmental health authority. Regulations and inspection ensure the use of approved equipment, good standards of hygiene and safety, proper waste disposal and correct after-care advice. These precautions are especially important: poor practice can transmit HIV, AIDS and hepatitis. Find qualified professionals in the *Yellow Pages*, through your local environmental health authority, or by a friend's recommendation. Never risk having these procedures done by an amateur or an unregistered person.

Piercing

The ear lobe

The basic pierced hole in each *ear lobe* makes wearing earrings comfortable and convenient. Many beauty salons and pharmacies offer quick, safe ear-piercing, using a 'gun' that shoots stud earrings into the lobes. Pain is minimal. Gold or gold-plated studs must be used; other metals can cause irritation or infection.

Afterwards, to prevent the holes from healing closed, you must leave the same stud earrings in place for six weeks. Follow the steps below prevent infection.

- Cleanse by wiping a liquid antiseptic over the front and back of the ear lobe twice a day; wash hands first.
- Each time you cleanse, turn the studs to prevent the hole closing – but otherwise do not touch or twiddle the studs.
- Avoid letting shampoo, soap, styling aids, fragrance, deodorant spray get on the ear lobes, and avoid swimming.
- Some tenderness is normal, but if the lobe becomes swollen or red, rinse the area frequently with boiled lukewarm salt water; see a doctor if it does not improve.

Multi-hole ear-piercing and nose-piercing

Two or three holes on the lobe, or one to a dozen on the upper, outer curved lip of the ear are not unusual. Nose-piercing is also popular. Both require the same basic care as basic ear-piercing.

Other parts of the body

Nipple and navel piercings require you to shower (not bath), to cleanse the piercing twice daily as above, and at nights to wear a T-shirt or a dressing over the wound until it's settled. If you venture into this kind of piercing be very careful about the skill of the practitioner and about aftercare and infection.

If you change your mind

If you want to back out while the piercing is still healing you must remove the stud and continue to care for the wound as described above. You may be left with a scar. If you change your mind after healing or even years later the hole will probably remain, or tissue may fill it in, making a scar.

Tattoos

From a tender little rose by your ankle to a dramatic serpent round your waist, a tattoo may tempt you as the ultimate individualist's style statement. Think it through thoroughly: a tattoo is a lifetime commitment. Only dermabrasion, skin peeling, laser treatment or surgery can remove it, perhaps only partially, often leaving an unattractive scar. It involves a bit of pain, too, and, like piercing, a risk of infection. You may not be welcome as a blood donor if you have a tattoo, because disreputable tattooists can transmit HIV, AIDS and hepatitis via their equipment. If you still want to consider it, here are some guidelines.

- Find a registered professional tattoo artist, as described above. Legally, he (usually he) cannot tattoo anyone under the age of 18.
- Visit the tattoo artist on a busy Saturday, look at the tattoo art on display and at the tattoos he's done on people waiting to be tattooed (they'll usually be keen to show you). Watch the artist at work. The studio should be clean and tidy. If you like the general feel of things, chat with the artist about the tattoo you'd like.

What design where?

Anything goes; as well as your own ideas, ask the tattooist about others – styles vary from one tattoo artist to another. Consider how often you want to flaunt your tattoo: intimate occasions only (hip, waist, buttock)? public view (ankle, wrist)? in between (shoulder, thigh)? Most professional tattoo artists will not tattoo hands, face or neck.

What happens?

The design is put on the skin with a transfer. The tattoo artist draws along the lines with a machine not unlike a small sewing machine which injects ink under the skin. Tattoo artists use various shapes and numbers of needles for different jobs, like painters use brushes.

How does it feel?

The tattoo procedure does hurt, but more in the order of annoyance than true pain. Areas close to bones (ankle, rib cage, spine) hurt more than fleshier places (upper arm, shoulder, thigh). The needle causes superficial blood flow.

What about afterwards?

Care is similar as for piercing, with the difference that a scab forms after two or three days. The tattoo should heal in eight to ten days.

Permanent eyeliner, lipliner and eyebrow colour

Cosmetic surgery clinics and some specialist beauty salons offer permanent or semi-permanent under-skin colouring. Sometimes called micropigmentation, it uses an electric needle to inject tiny dots of pigment into the skin, but it does not penetrate as deep as tattooing. The colouring is matched to your natural colouring to give definition where you would normally use make-up for the same purpose. Particularly useful for people with pale lashes or sparse or missing eyebrows, it's subtle – you may still want to wear make-up – but permanent for five years or so.

PERMANENT BEAUTY CHANGE CHECKLIST

- Do your homework and fieldwork. Gather information and examine your hopes and motives.
- Take your time. It's your body, and your lifetime to live with this permanent change.
- Heed your gut instinct. In the end, only you can decide.

12
INSIDE THE BEAUTY BUSINESS

When you're buying a body lotion or considering an eyeshadow, have you ever paused to wonder how the product came into being? Every one of these has a long chain of people, companies, science, technology, regulations and showmanship behind it. You'll be a better-informed consumer if you know a bit of the inside story – it's fascinating.

The cradle of all cosmetics and healing remedies was the kitchen of the wise woman herbalist. But around the turn of the 19th century two extraordinary, canny women, Helena Rubinstein and Elizabeth Arden, brewed home-made skin-care recipes to sell and to use in their own treatment salons. Both women soon employed chemists to augment their efforts. By the 1920s these two great rivals had thriving international businesses, and even today their names and genius thrive on. What they had simultaneously discovered was the power of marketing: knowing what women need and wish for; providing an effective, safe product to meet those needs and wishes; presenting the needed, wished-for product by naming and packaging it, making it known, making it available. The birth of a new product still works this way, only on a multi-layered, mega basis.

How a product is born

Conception

It's a toss-up whether the twinkle in the eye for a beauty product occurs in the chemists' laboratory, the marketing department or the packaging design studio. Some products arise because a scientist discovers a new or improved ingredient that has a desirable effect – say skin-exfoliating, alpha-hydroxy fruit acids in a cream that simultaneously moisturises.

Other products are created because a marketing expert discovers that consumers have an unmet need or desire. This discovery is based on studies of trends in the consumer population and sales of existing products. A new range of glossy lipsticks might come about like this: the post Second World War baby-boom population bulge resonates as the original babyboomers (now in their early fifties) have children who are now in their early twenties; as teens these children wore lip gloss ... now they're growing more sophisticated, but they still like gloss; conclusion – a glossy lipstick will appeal to this market segment. It must be inexpensive, because they're used to low-priced lipgloss and they are not earning huge amounts of money.

Beauty products also originate from packaging engineers who may initiate ideas or put heads together with chemists and marketing executives. Much of a product's usefulness and appeal lies in its delivery, which depends as much on the bottle, jar, tube, valve, applicator, neck opening, etc. as on the mix of ingredients. Styling mousse, after all, is basically creamy setting lotion with plasticisers in it; reformulated and pressurised by aerosol, it foams for easy, satisfying application.

Development

Once a product is conceived it goes into development. A small pilot batch is made up and put into plain containers. Products from the batch go off in various directions ...

1 To the marketing department creative team, either in-house or through an agency, for a name, graphics, image. These must convey what the product is and, equally important, what the wish, dream or mood appeal is. Lipcolour that lasts? Skincare if you have oily breakout?
2 To the packaging engineers for interpretation of design into reality for the shop shelf, for use, for practicalities of supply and production. Does the shampoo look appealing through the plastic? Will the blusher compact close and open efficiently?
3 Back in the marketing department business minds are working out

INSIDE THE HEALTH AND BEAUTY BUSINESS

quantities, pricing, advertising and promotion budgets. Do we supply all six shades of the new blusher in equal amounts? What are the actual costs of ingredients and packaging?

4 Before long, at the factory, production engineers work with the cosmetic chemists and packaging engineers to order ingredients in bulk, pilot production runs, schedule the use of huge, stainless steel vats, adapt filling, labelling and shrink-wrapping machines.

5 At last development comes to a crescendo with the product launch co-ordinated by the marketing department: advertising, promotional items, press releases and events, sales department training and distribution networks reveal the product to retailers, media and the public.

6 Meanwhile, throughout development, starting with that first pilot batch, a cosmetic product undergoes batteries of tests to ensure:
- stability – it's heated in ovens and chilled in refrigerators to simulate climate, shipping, shelf-life and consumer-use excesses.
- purity – it's 'challenged' in a petri dish or by having certain bacteria mixed with it, to see if it will make too happy an environment for moulds or other unpleasantries. This simulates the fact that a user may take a year to finish off a product, which amounts to a year of possible contamination by less-than-sterile fingers.
- performance and safety – it may be tested on paid volunteers or on animals (more on this below). Does it indeed smooth the skin or colour the hair or last twice as long as other products? Excessive claims are not allowed, and safety in use is essential.
- package compatability – the product is used and left to stand to be sure that oils, alcohols, plastics or other ingredients don't ruinously interact with the plastics, print, paper or other package materials.
- appeal – market testing puts the product before panels of the ideal consumer and/or sells it in a limited geographical area to be sure the whole concept – name, design, image and performance – appeals.
- quality control – technicians in the factory take random samples of every production batch (every batch is numbered and recorded). These are kept for tests to ensure purity and stability, and for evaluation should there be a consumer safety complaint.

By the time a product reaches you it's had quite a life. In the best scenario, it makes your beauty wish come true!

Confronting beauty issues

Animal testing and alternatives

Your skin is vital and living, and it has many crucial functions. Not only an organ of protection and regulation, it also can transmit substances into the body. You must be sure, and anyone who makes cosmetics must be sure, that products that touch the skin are safe to use, not only once but daily — this is the reason for testing ingredients and products on animals. How would you feel about a severe skin rash, eye irritation, mouth ulcers, blindness, hair loss, skin cancer, defects to your unborn children or similar from use of a cosmetic product? Did you know that numerous Elizabethan beauties died of lead poisoning from the white face make-up they wore? Mice, rabbits, rats, guinea pigs ... is it fair to shave them to patch test creams, to inject collagen, to feed them lipstick, to drip shampoo in their eyes? Fair, no, but necessary to protect humans, scientists insist.

We could wish for alternatives to animal testing, and there are some. Humans in prison are sometimes asked to try out new products. Cosmetics-makers or agencies may pay volunteers to use products. One company even paid a convent of nuns to use a cream on their virgin (to cosmetics) skin. Many companies today test on humans only and clearly state that no animal testing has occurred.

However, it's not quite as simple as this. It is the nature of science, not cosmetics, that requires animal testing. Legally and scientifically the word 'cosmetics' means hygiene items such as toothpaste, soap and deodorant as well as beautifiers such as lipsticks, mascara and moisturiser. We would not today have fluoride toothpaste, anti-dandruff shampoo or sunscreens if it were not for animal testing. Laws don't specifically state that products must be animal tested – it's just that they must be proven not to be harmful. But scientists advise the government regulators, and scientific method generally admits only data from animal tests.

Developmental and future possible alternatives acceptable to scientific standards include test-tube cell-culture (*in vitro*) — human or animal cells are grown in laboratories and their response to the product or ingredient indicates safety or toxicity. Computer analysis of chemical components and computers programmed to virtual human response are also possibilities.

The truth is all ingredients have been tested at some time, even if they are now known to be safe and are no longer animal tested. In actuality, there is an unwritten parenthesis after the words 'not tested' saying 'in the last five years' or 'since 1985'. Most beauty products are made from some of the 6,000 ingredients on the European Union's INCI list (pronounced 'inky', it stands for International Nomenclature for Cosmetic Ingredients). A further refinement, used on both sides of the Atlantic, is the GRAS list (Generally Regarded as Safe) – ingredients long-known and scientifically accepted as harmless in cosmetics.

If animal testing worries you, be wary, and read label wording carefully. While a company may not animal test the final product, it may animal test some of the ingredients. Also, some manufacturers may not animal test, but they may buy ingredients from suppliers who conduct animal tests. Finally, although a company can ask, it may not know for sure if some ingredients it buys have been animal tested or not.

Last but not least, for your own safety, most governments insist that certain products and ingredients, and certainly any that are radically new, are tested scientifically, which usually means on animals, to be proven safe for human use. So there will always be some animal testing of some cosmetic products.

What can you do?

In ascending order of commitment:

- Use products from reputable firms, confident in their state-of-the-art safety.
- Look for products and ingredients labelled as not tested on animals, or for products labelled as vegetarian (produced without killing or harming animals) or even vegan (using no animal products, not even eggs, honey, milk, etc).
- Volunteer to an animal protection society or a cosmetics company to be a human test subject.
- Write to manufacturers expressing your concerns.
- Make your own products from foodstuffs (olive oil, lemon juice, etc).
- Give up grooming and cosmetics entirely?

Natural products, how natural?

'Natural' is a word that has come to mean all good things – 'green' consciousness, health-giving, un-hyped, superior to contemporary technology, subtle, gentle, pure, good-old-days. Written on the label of a conditioner or tonic it makes you think: good stuff! Think again. Nettles are natural, and they sting. Primroses can give a rash. Yew and foxglove are natural, and they can kill. Crude oil emerges naturally from the earth, arsenic is a natural element. Beyond this, think for a moment about what's unnatural: cutting your hair, eating at a table with a knife and fork, reading this book – 'natural' isn't the only good way to be. So when you see the word 'natural' attached to a product, be aware that it can mean almost anything:

- The minimum: ingredients include a pinch of camomile or other herbs (also called botanicals).
- The maximum: ingredients use no synthetics (generally this means no petrochemicals; soya, palm, almond, avocado, grapeseed or other botanical oils are used instead of paraffin-based mineral oils).
- Ingredients may or may not use animal products or by-products such as collagen, tallow, lanolin, bee jelly.
- Other environmentally conscious 'buzz words' (hypo-allergenic, fragrance-free, dermatologically tested, cruelty-free, not tested on animals) may imply 'natural' – or 'natural' may imply these things.
- The day is dawning when the line between natural and technological is blurred. Where food and drugs break ground, cosmetics will soon follow: today protein meat substitutes are grown and harvested, salmon are farmed, genetic engineering allows production of insulin. At least one major cosmetics-maker currently grows tiny yeasts in giant vats for a bio-engineered safe and sophisticated skin cream.

What to do?

- Read and interpret labels closely.
- Ask questions of sales people or manufacturers.
- Grow and make your own beauty aids if you are really concerned.

Miracle claims – how deep is skin deep?

Some companies make vague and extraordinary claims for the effectiveness of their products, particularly skincare. Do you ever get the feeling you're being bamboozled? The truth is, some products are even more effective than they claim to be.

Legally, cosmetic products can only treat the epidermis; anything that has an effect on the dermis (the skin's deeper living layer, see

Chapter 4) should be classified as a drug. Many new-generation skin products, however, contain ingredients that genuinely improve the look and feel of skin not only by their action on the epidermis, but also by penetrating and acting at a deeper layer. Take as examples three 'anti-ageing' ingredients: AHAs, antioxidants, and tretinoin.

Alpha-hydroxy acids AHAs are thought to work by speeding up the shedding of the top epidermal layers. However, recent dermatological tests showed that they measurably increase skin thickness, water-holding ability and elastin resilience – in other words, they make skin act and look more youthful.

Antioxidants These, particularly vitamins E and C, theoretically prevent skin-cell damage by de-fusing free radicals caused by UV rays, pollution and normal metabolism. They may even help skin-cell immunity, reducing the risk of cancer. For one product, a dermatological photograph shows dramatically less-wrinkled skin after use of an antioxidant treatment.

Tretinoin An active ingredient related to vitamin A, tretinoin is thought to act by mildly irritating the epidermis or by activating receptors that control skin protein production. Either way (or both) it repairs fine wrinkles, fades age spots, smooths the skin.

Under the microscope and even, to various degrees, to the naked eye, the visible effects of all three are known – they really do help ageing skin. The mechanisms of all three are still under scientific investigation. But the last is a drug, and the first two are cosmetics. Tretinoin, contained in Ortho Pharmaceutical's product Renova (in the USA; in Britain it's called Retinova) is the first prescription-only wrinkle treatment approved by the US Food and Drug Administration (FDA). It cost many millions of pounds to run the massive clinical trials required for FDA approval.

Why haven't companies put AHAs and antioxidants in for FDA approval? Because as cosmetics – tested as safe and effective but not tested to drug-approval levels – there's no huge scientific trials cost. What's more, there's wider marketing freedom for cosmetics; drugs have stringent legal advertising limits. Cosmetics' claims are restricted, too, but advertisements can make the vague and pretty promises that are forbidden to medical science. The only fly in this ointment is that the claim made for a bonafide active cosmetic treatment sounds much the same as a simple but ordinary product.

What to do?

- Buy from reputable companies.
- Read carefully about new products in health and beauty pages.
- If you're seriously interested, study dermatology.
- Take all claims with a pinch of salt.
- Remember, your health, lifestyle, regular basic skincare and sunscreens are more important to your looks than any 'miracle' cream.

Fear of the dragon lady – surviving the sales pitch

Are you daunted by the gauntlet of impeccably groomed, uniformed, sometimes over-madeup women who grace department store beauty counters? There they hover, amid glowing lighting, gleaming trays, polished glass. The aim of all this showmanship is to make you feel privileged and pampered. If, instead, you feel intimidated and fear that you'll be persuaded to buy too much, here's how to cope:

- Keep a firm beauty need in mind: spots, dry skin, a new lipstick, something specific.
- Set a budget in advance – and if you feel tempted or pressured, announce your strict budget to the salesperson.
- Be knowledgeable, so she can't blind you with science. Know your skin type and your personal needs, read health and beauty magazines so you know the latest jargon.
- Be willing to learn from the salesperson; if what she tells you sounds convincing it could be true. She has had weeks of training, and she has the experience of helping lots of people every day.
- Don't feel obliged to overspend after having a free make-up or facial – it's the company's risk that you won't buy.
- Be cautious about linked products – some are genuine, like toner after cleansing lotion, some are redundant, like throat cream on top of anti-wrinkle cream. Refuse to buy a near substitute if they don't have what you want; ask to order your product. A salesperson may push a product on you if it's earning her a bonus or if she's out of stock of what you want.
- Develop a relationship with the salesperson. She'll be delighted to have a regular customer and you can begin to rely on her advice.
- If you don't like being served this way buy off the shelf from pharmacies, supermarkets or department store toiletries departments. The quality is just fine, even if the packages and prices are less glitzy.

TAKE ADVANTAGE OF COSMETICS COMPANIES' NEEDS AND FEARS

- Promotional items, trial sizes, bonus sizes, two-for-the-price-of-one, tote bags and T-shirts and handy kits containing products — they're great buys! Companies usually lose their normal profits on these, just to reward faithful customers or to win new ones. They hope you'll return to buy their normal items — but that's entirely up to you.
- Product complaints. If a product irritates your skin, a package or applicator is damaged or you have any other genuine complaint, write to the cosmetic company about it. Believe me, manufacturers care intensely that their products are safe and well presented – their whole image may be at stake. You will probably get a letter of apology and a new or replacement product or a voucher in return.

  How to go about it: explain the problem, enclose the product (sales slip, too, if you still have it). Most products have a company address on the package, some even have customer telephone lines; you can also take it back to the shop. Obviously, you should make only legitimate complaints and do it before you've used the product to its last drop.

Product lowdown: a glossary of ingredients

Read the ingredients label on a beauty product and what do you see? A few things you can recognise, like paraffin oil (refined petroleum oil), aqua (water – there's a lot of it in many products), beeswax, jojoba oil, aloe vera extract, kaolin (clay), grapeseed oil... but the number of mysterious or jaw-breaking scientific names on most lists is daunting – just what are they, what do they do? To crack the code totally you need a chemist's bible, such as *Harry's Cosmeticology*, available in technical libraries. Meanwhile, here's a random glossary of 20 ingredients you'll find in many beauty products.

Ingredient	Function
Allantoin	healing agent
BHA, BHT (Butylated Hydroxyanisole or Hydroxyoluene)	preservatives
Cetyl alcohol	emulsifying agent, often in creams
Carnauba	very hard vegetable wax for firming lipstick
FD&C Blue No 1 Aluminium Lake	blue pigment; Aluminium Lakes are good for translucent colour
Imidazolidinyl urea	preservative, stabiliser, humectant
Iron oxides	black, red or yellow pigments
Isopropol palmitate	a water-free, water-resistant liquid to help application of a product
Glycerin	humectant, for moisture attraction and retention
Glyceryl ricinoleate (castor oil)	dispenses pigment and gives gloss, usually in lipsticks
Methylcellulose	film-forming material
Methylchlorothymol	preservative
Methylparaben (also Ethyl-, Butyl-, Propyl-)	parabens are preservatives
Panthenol	vitamin B
Polyethylene	waterproofing agent
Sodium carbomer	carbomers are thickening agents, for ease of product application
Sodium lauryl sulphate	surface acting agent, e.g. the foam in shampoo
Sorbitol	emollient, humectant, and aids application
Titanium dioxide	white pigment used to achieve pink shades and for opacity of coverage
Tocopherol	vitamin E, an antioxidant (preservative)

Beauty futures

What's in store for healthy beauty in the new millennium? More of the same, more refined, more advanced. Science is always pushing the frontiers of knowledge, and the world of beauty will adapt discoveries. New computer and material technologies multiply the possibilities. Even the past is helping the future, with the discovery and validation of 'new' old plants, tribal wisdom, ancient lore.

But perhaps beauty lies in your own future. If you'd like to be more informed about healthy beauty and wellbeing, look to adult education and holistic health centres for courses on anatomy and physiology, nutrition, aromatherapy, reflexology, herbalism, massage, grooming, assertiveness, etc. If you're hooked on feeling good and looking good and if you like the idea of helping others to do the same, perhaps you'd like a career in the field. There's potential for a wide range of skills, interests, ages and levels of education.

Your own beauty future: could you be a beauty business insider?

Here are some career possibilities, in random order:

- Hairdresser – cutting, styling, colouring, perming.
- Trichologist – hair and scalp health specialist.
- Beauty consultant – salesperson for a cosmetic company, usually working in a store, possibly home sales. Trained by the company.
- Beauty therapist – facials, bodycare, nailcare, make-up.
- Electrologist – hair removal, small vein diathermy.
- Aromatherapist – massage and use of essential oils.
- Make-up artist – employed by a salon or cosmetic company or freelance; work on clients and give demonstrations.
- Post-surgical/remedial make-up counsellor – for a clinic or hospital.
- Fitness leader – from aerobics, step training and weights to yoga and tai chi, in a gym, leisure classes, clinic or as a personal trainer.
- Complementary medicine practitioner – improving wellbeing through homoeopathy, herbalism, osteopathy, Alexander Technique, reflexology, acupuncture, others.
- Counsellor – improving wellbeing and confidence through talking.
- Colour and wardrobe consultant – analysing colour suitability, body image, giving dress guidance. Trained by the company.

All of the above involve personal contact, many of them require hands-on contact, so you need a nurturing urge and you have to be good with people. You also have to maintain your own good looks and wellbeing in order to give clients confidence. Except where mentioned, most of the above require training and qualifications, but none require a university degree. Many are suitable for young people, and they can make good mid-life career changes.

If you'd like to be a creator, mover, shaker or shaper of beauty consider the areas listed below. Some will appeal to numerate and technically-minded people, others to creative or communicative types. Many of the jobs here require some kind of further or higher education.

- Chemist – analysing, inventing, testing products.
- Engineer – package design, package and product production.
- Marketing – masterminding the creation of a product.
- Sales – working with retailers to distribute products.
- Graphic artist – creating the look of products, advertising, etc.
- Photographer – for print or screen: shooting models or still-lifes for ads, promotional materials or magazines.
- Stylist – arranging clothes, props for photography or video/filming.
- Make-up artist – specialising beyond client work for the ins and outs of photography and shows.
- Hair stylist – as for specialist make-up artist.
- Fashion design/colour consultant – predicting consumer directions and colour trends for manufacturers.
- Journalist/beauty editor – covering health and beauty news for magazines, newspapers, trade. Often responsible for briefing and selecting the cover photos of women's and fashion magazines.
- Copywriter – writing the words of ads, scripts, slogans, names, instructions, promotional material
- Public relations – communicating product news to the media; either in-house at a cosmetics company or at an agency.
- Nurse, doctor, dentist, chiropodist, pharmacist – the health fields are the ultimate in serious personal care, and medical and paramedical qualifications are highly valued in the cosmetics industry.

Some variations on the theme: extremely difficult to get into, but if you're star-struck and determined ...

- Model – no degree needed! If you think you have the looks (and stamina), get to know names of reputable modelling agencies by

reading magazines (or write to magazines). Write or telephone to ask how they want to be approached. Usually you need to build up a portfolio of professional photographs of yourself; you could start by befriending a want-to-be fashion/beauty photographer.
- Film, television, video or stage hair stylist or make-up artist – you usually need both hair and make-up skills, plus training so you know about creating looks for historical periods, blood and gore, fantasy, etc. Be prepared to travel and to work in unglamorous conditions. Gain early experience by working in amateur theatre.

Step by step: how to begin your beauty future

Step 1 Gather information by talking to beauty workers you encounter (in shops, at salons and clinics) – ask them how they got started.

Step 2 Enquire at local libraries and colleges.

Step 3 Ask careers advice centres and employment bureaux if they know of local training opportunities, sometimes free or funded by government schemes. You might want to plunge right in with a beginner's position at a local beauty company, if there is one, although you'll eventually need training to progress.

Step 4 Write with enquiries to cosmetic companies and professional organisations (see Resources at the back of this book).

Step 5 From the information gathered, consider what training and possible licensing you'll need; some jobs require one- or two-year training courses, some need higher education diplomas or degrees or technical qualifications, some require work placement or apprenticeship. Weigh the cost and time it will take, the income you can earn and the satisfaction you'll get.

MIRROR, MIRROR

Welcome! At the completion of this book I hope you feel that you're now something of a beauty insider, free to claim your own healthy, liveable good looks and personal style. Enjoy making the most of yourself and your know-how. This isn't the end but the beginning.

RESOURCES

Books

Ageless Ageing, The Natural Way to Stay Young, Leslie Kenton, Century Arrow ISBN 0 09 946690 2

Basic Hairdressing, A Coursebook for NVQ Level 2, Stephanie Henderson, Stanley Thornes Publishers ISBN 0 7487 2238 6

Careers in Hairdressing and Beauty Therapy, Alexa Stace, Kogan Page ISBN 0 7494 1060 4

Harry's Cosmeticology, edited by JB Wilkinson and RJ Moore, George Godwin ISBN 0 7114 5679 8

A Practical Guide to Beauty Therapy for NVQ Level 2, Janet Simms, Stanley Thornes Publishers ISBN 0 7487 1508 8

Teach Yourself Alexander Technique, Richard Craze, Hodder & Stoughton ISBN 0 340 64819 8

Teach Yourself Aromatherapy, Denise Brown, Hodder & Stoughton ISBN 0 340 65491 0

Teach Yourself Healthy Eating, Wendy Doyle, Hodder & Stoughton ISBN 0 340 57257 4

Teach Yourself Managing Stress, Terry Looker and Olga Gregson, Hodder & Stoughton ISBN 0 340 66376 6

Help/information organisations

These are listed for the United Kingdom only; include a stamped, self-addressed envelope (SAE) with your enquiry. In other countries, read newspaper and magazine beauty and health articles to discover similar organisations; also try books, libraries, *Yellow Pages*, health and beauty clinics/salons and your doctor.

Action on Smoking and Health (ASH), Devon House, 12–15 Dartmouth Street, London SW1H 9BL. *Help on giving up smoking*

Amarant Trust, Grant House, 56–60 St John Street, London EC1M 4DT. *Menopause and HRT information and clinic*

British Association for Aesthetic Plastic Surgeons, Royal College of Surgeons, 35–43 Lincoln's Inn Fields, London WC2 3PN. *List of registered surgeons for cosmetic medical treatment*

British Dental Health Foundation, Eastland Court, St Peter's Road, Rugby, Warks CV21 3QP. *Information on cosmetic dentistry and other aspects of dental care*

Brook Advisory Centres, 165 Grays Inn Road, London, WC1X 8UD. Tel: 0171 713 9000. Numerous locations. *Advice and counselling on emotional and sexual problems*

Changing Faces, 1 & 2 Junction Mews, Paddington, London W2 1PN. *Disfigurement counselling*

Institute for Complementary Medicine, PO Box 194, London SE16 1QZ. *Include two, loose, first class stamps for information on therapies and practitioners in your area*

Weight Watchers UK Ltd., Kidswell Park House, Kidswell Park Drive, Maidenhead, Berks SL6 8YT. *For information and programmes.*

Women's Nutritional Advisory Service, PO Box 268, Lewes, East Sussex BN7 2QN. *Include four, loose, first class stamps with your specific enquiry on PMS, menopause or other health concerns*

Career training/professional organisations

United Kingdom
British Association of Beauty Therapy and Cosmetology (BABTAC), Parabola House, Parabola Road, Cheltenham, Gloucester GL50 3AH

Hairdressing Training Board, 3 Chequer Road, Doncaster DN1 2AA

Society of Cosmetic Scientists, GT House, 24–26 Rothesay Road, Luton, Bedforshire LU1 1QX

United States
National Cosmetology Association, Esthetics Division, 3510 Olive Street, St Louis, Missouri 63103

Canada
Canadian International Esthetics Associations, 824–470 Granville Street, Vancouver BC V6V 1VS

Australia
The Australian Federation of Aestheticians and Beauty Therapists, Box 2078 GPO Brisbane 4001

INDEX

acid–alkaline balance 41, 62, 102, 115, 130
acne 52, 164
aerobic 29–30
African, Afro-Caribbean 38, 42, 46, 50, 58, 68, 72, 96, 103, 116, 143
ageing skin 179 (and *see* mature)
ages and stages 9, 43, 52–3, 83–4, 93, 104, 117, 149–53, 163
AHAs 49, 179
Alexander Technique 8, 158, 160, 183
alopecia 69
anaerobic 30–2
animal testing 176
Asian 38, 42, 44, 50, 58, 72, 116, 142, 143
assessment (*see* self-assessment)
birthmarks 53, 117, 163
Black, see African/Afro-Caribbean
blackheads 51
bone strength 30, 35, 153, 154
breasts 20, 30, 80, 140–1, 151, 154, 166
caffeine 18, 24, 158
cardiovascular 12
cellulite 13, 140
childbirth (*see* pregnancy)
circulation 12, 29, 140
collagen 41, 49, 165, 178
complementary medicine 17, 158, 159, 183
constipation 13, 16
contraception 150–1
dandruff 67–8
diathermy 53, 163, 183
electrical treatment 56, 140, 142
electrolysis 53, 142, 163, 183
excess hair (*see* hair)
exercise routines 29–34
eyebrows 112, 118–9, 122
eyeglasses 126
face shapes 76, 90–2
facial hair 53
fats 16, 20–1
fibre 16, 21
free radicals 42, 179
hair, chemical safety 101
hair cuts 67, 94–7
hair, excess of 141
hair, loss of 68–9
hormones 9, 12, 13-14, 42, 60, 69, 131, 140, 147, 149–53, 159
humectant 41, 47, 49
immune system 14, 148–9, 160
keratin 58, 61–2, 98, 102, 133
Latina 38, 42, 116, 143
lymph, lymphatic system 14, 41, 55, 56, 140, 148, 156
massage, self 156–7
mature health and beauty 9, 42–3, 53, 83–4, 93, 117, 152–3, 154

Mediterranean 38, 42, 142
melanin 38, 42, 60, 143
menopause 30, 52, 69, 152–3, 154
menstruation 149–51
metabolism 7, 9, 12, 16, 41, 159
microcirculation 36, 48, 49, 55, 56, 60, 71, 148
minerals 16–17, 21, 158
moles 53, 145, 163
muscles 28–9
nutrients 12, 14, 15–17, 21, 26, 71
Oriental 38, 58, 72
osteopath 8, 158, 160
oxygenation 12, 35
pH (*see* acid/alkaline)
photographic make-up 128
posture 7–8, 32, 159
pregnancy 9, 36, 69, 83, 151–2, 163
premenstrual syndrome, PMS, PMT 150–1, 152, 158, 159
product claims 177–9
rescue 107, 129
rosacea 52
scars 53, 117
seasons of colour 72–5, 116
sebum 39, 41, 42, 58, 59, 65
self-assessments 5, 38–9, 57–9, 72–4, 76–8, 90–4
sensitive skin 50
sex 36–7, 150, 154, 155, 159
shopping 85–6, 180–1
smoking 36, 154
split ends 59, 67
step-by-steps 84–5, 119–25, 135–6, 138
stress 32, 146–8, 156–9
style, types of 81–3, 108–9
style, 20th century 88
sugar 19–20
sun 42, 47, 110, 142–4
suppleness 32–4
teenage health and beauty 16, 42, 52, 83, 149–50, 155, 163
television appearance 128
thinning hair 68–9
toxins 12, 13, 18, 48, 49, 140, 149
tretinoin 179
trichologist 70, 183
troubled skin 51–2
UV rays (*see* sun)
vaginal care 36, 80, 139, 152, 154–6
varicose veins 164
visual laws 78–9
vitamins 16–17, 21, 158
water 16, 18
Weight Watchers 7, 18
white hair 68, 104
whitehead 52